HUMAN BANK™

HUMAN BANK™

The Wise Investor

Michael J. Smith

Author's Note on Copyright & Ethical Sharing

This book is the result of years of reflection, research, and lived experience. It is my heartfelt desire that it blesses, empowers, and enriches your life.

I kindly ask that you respect the copyright of this work. No part of this publication may be reproduced, stored in a retrieval system, or transmitted in any form or by any means—electronic, mechanical, photocopying, recording, or otherwise—without the prior written permission of the publisher, except in the case of brief quotations used in reviews or articles.

If you found this book valuable, the best way to honour its message is by sharing a link to purchase it legally or encouraging others to support the work directly.

If you would like to use this content in a course, community, or organisation, I would love to connect—please reach out via the contact details provided.

Thank you for your integrity and support in protecting and sharing the message of the Human Bank™.

Trademark Notice

Human Bank™ is a trademark of **Human Profit Pty Ltd**.

All rights reserved. This name, concept, and associated materials may not be used in connection with any product or service not authorised by the author, in any manner likely to cause confusion among readers or participants.

Scripture Acknowledgement

All Scripture quotations, unless otherwise noted, are taken from the **ESV Bible (The Holy Bible, English Standard Version)**, © Crossway, a publishing ministry of Good News Publishers. Used by permission. All rights reserved.

First Edition – June 2025
ISBN: eBook: 978-0-6487235-0-9   Paperback: 978-0-6487235-1-6
Cover Design: Michael Smith   **Cover Image:** Antonio Lapa
Published by: Human Profit Pty Ltd **Printed by:** IngramSpark

For permissions or speaking engagements, contact: www.humanbank.life

I dedicate this book to my Heavenly Father and to all people of the world, that they may find eternal life in Him.

Acknowledgements

Thank You, Heavenly Father, for Your everlasting love—for all You have done and been for me, for inspiring and helping me write this book. I am forever grateful. May it be for Your glory!

To my son, Samuel—thank you for who you are: an amazing young man. You are a gift. Thank you for helping with this book and inspiring a second.

To Robin and Riti—thank you for your friendship and for the hours sown into the soil of this book. Today, we see the fruit.

To Justin and Bec—what a lifeline! Thank you for stepping in at a critical time and helping shape the final words with clarity and grace.

To Elie and Sandy—all I can say is, you made this possible. Thank you for making a way for me to write—for your obedience, sacrifice, and endless service to others.

To Kuya Dan and Ate Tanette—thank you for the years of faithfulness, prayer, love, and support on the journey. I thank God for you.

To my family and parents, Roger and Lesley—you are not able to see this book, but I see you in it. Thank you for your love, support, sacrifice, and belief you invested in me.

To all who have prayed, helped, or inspired me and the *Human Bank* book—thank you.

God bless you. And the journey continues—**the journey to invest for life that is true life.**

Contents

Introduction

As I sit here and pen these words, I reflect on the global wellbeing crisis. A crisis we see only in part, yet feel deeply. It is a crisis of physical, emotional, relational, mental, and soul wellbeing. People are stretched thin, weighed down by stress, burned out, anxious, fearful, restless for peace, longing for love, searching for meaning and struggling to find hope. People are empty.

We all have modes and methods of coping; some healthy, some unhealthy, some constructive and some destructive. People struggle to navigate the demands and crises of life, work, relationships and family. Most of all, people search for answers to deeper, soul-related questions like "who am I?" and "what am I here for?" "What is the meaning of life, and how do I get peace?"

Some readers may put down this book because they do not want to know God's love or the eternal life He offers to all. It is a confronting book — one that challenges our decisions and exposes how the devil steals from our lives. That is your choice, but if I truly desire to help people prosper in life, I need to address every aspect of life, including the spiritual. Then it is up to the individual reader to decide what they do from there. The choices you make will determine your future. I hope and pray your path is one that leads to true life!

My story

I grew up in the south-west suburbs of Sydney in government housing, in an area with one of the highest crime rates. Social dysfunction, negativity, and hopelessness were rampant. I lived with my parents, my eldest brother, and our pet dog, Sooty.

My parents separated when I was five years old, and that began a new and difficult season. All I can say is that it felt like evil darkness was pursuing me to damage and overtake my life.

I was in survival mode during my primary school years, which saw my education and development slow to a crawl. My big brother was protective and looked out for me. Crime, drugs, and violence were all around — yet I chose not to pursue that path.

Michael J. Smith

Dad took us to church regularly, for which I am eternally grateful (thank you). It was a light that helped me feel connected to God and to what is good in a dark world.

I was already behind when I went to high (secondary) school and didn't progress much during that time — just scraping through each year. I don't know how. I didn't understand maths or English. My English was basic, my grammar very limited, and my vocabulary even more so. It most likely didn't improve much.

I left school at the age of 16 to work as a kitchen hand scrubbing pots, and my working career began.

I moved to the Northern Beaches at the age of 19 to be with close friends I had grown up with, and I worked at an Italian restaurant. The owners were very entrepreneurial, and one day I realised there was more to life than four walls and a kitchen.

So, at the age of 20, I studied Asia-Pacific Marketing at college (the only option available with my level of education). I desired more and pursued it — despite my limited education and capacity.

Me writing this book is not a testament to my literary brilliance, but to the grace and enablement of God — and the good editors who supported the process.

I became a follower of Jesus at the age of 23. At the time, I was a partner in a successful business. I was also one of the most arrogant, self-centred, prideful people you could meet. It was all about money, status, and appearance. Anything that helped to cover up all my insecurities and lack of identity.

Then, on a Friday night in November, I experienced the love of God. He took me on a journey of discovery and healing, a deep healing of my heart, emotions, and soul. It was a painful journey but one that brought new life, peace, and restoration. I came to see myself as very one dimensional; my only concern was my physical appearance, with little or no concern for the other things necessary to have a whole life. Over time, I came to realise that living a satisfying and meaningful life requires giving attention to five key areas:

Physically wellbeing - this obviously refers to physical health, diet, and exercise. Good physical wellbeing empowers us to live longer, do more, think clearer, and directly impacts our mental health, too.

Emotional wellbeing - that is, understanding how I feel, how to manage my emotions, and how to invest in them so that I am emotionally healthy.

Relational wellbeing - the relationships in my life, what I am investing into them and what are they investing into me contribute to my relational and overall wellbeing. Am I relating and acting out of woundedness or wholeness? Am I relating out of pride, insecurities or anxieties? God took me on a journey of discovering an identity that was meaningful and fulfilling in Him.

Mental wellbeing - this is relating to thoughts, beliefs, and how we perceive the world. When we have emotional or psychological wounds, they profoundly affect how we see ourselves and the world around us. My own journey was one of transitioning from insecure, limited thinking regarding my place and purpose in the world to living a life of confidence, and greater purpose.

Soul wellbeing - the most important discovery is that every person has a soul. You may respond with surprise or scepticism as I once did, but it's true. What is the soul? It is not just a mystical term but relates to the spiritual, eternal aspect of our lives. Before I became a Christian, I lived what could be called by most peoples' definition a very immoral life. Yes, I did whatever I wanted, but I had this growing feeling of guilt, shame and condemnation which made me feel insecure. I didn't think I was a good person because I was doing bad things. This led to me trying to cover-up my inner turmoil with a continuous cycle of pleasure and escape, especially partying and drinking. When I became a Christian, I found forgiveness in God that took away my guilt, shame and condemnation. This profoundly affected my identity, as you can imagine. It started a new cycle of peace and rest. I came to realise that more than any other area, my spiritual health directly influenced my identity, passions and desires, will and intellect. When my soul was not healthy, it affected almost every other area of life.

As I walked my own journey toward healing, I developed an awareness of my whole life wellbeing. It quickly became apparent that all of us experience wellbeing issues, and I started to wonder how to help others invest in the areas briefly described above, known as the P.E.R.M.S areas of wellbeing. Through this experience, I developed the Human Profit concept and a wellbeing index that helped people measure their health and wellbeing. In 2009, businesses and organisations started using this wellbeing index, and it has been used to help hundreds of people. And so, the journey of the Human Bank™ began.

Michael J. Smith

ABC's of Human Bank

We live in a world that is overdrawn — filled with burnout, anxiety, loneliness, lack, hopelessness, addiction, and disconnection from God. The Human Bank™ reveals the root causes of these issues through a biblical lens and shows how to bring healing and restore profit and purpose.

Human Bank™ represents our whole-life wellbeing. By integrating economic theory with ancient Biblical truths, this book empowers us to assess, measure, and invest in our wellbeing, enabling us to truly prosper in the five areas of our Human Bank: physical, emotional, relational, mental, and soul. It is an evidence-based system that helps assess the positive and negative investments we make into our Human Banks and the impacts these have on our lives. The Human Bank™ is designed as a tool to help us grow in our whole life wellbeing and to avoid the pitfalls of poor wellbeing, so that we live the lives we were created for: profitable ones, full of meaning and recognised potential.

At the Core: A Spiritual Revelation

The Human Bank™ is rooted in three core truths:

1. God is the Source – He alone fills us with energy (life), joy, love, peace, and freedom.
2. Jesus is the Way – Through His sacrifice, we receive access to restored life and healing.
3. The Holy Spirit is the Power – He dwells in us to fill, renew, and transform our inner world.

Without God, our banks run dry. With God, our banks overflow.

"Beloved, I pray that you may prosper in all things and be in health, just as your soul prospers." — 3 John 1:2

Who is it for?

Although Human Profit was designed for businesses and organisations, the Human Bank™ is for everybody; after all, everyone has wellbeing. Every person, whether a teacher, student, athlete, office worker, parent, lawyer or artist has a need to flourish and prosper in life and we will need help on the journey in different ways at different times. This book is a tool in your hand to help you prosper in any (or all) of the H areas in which you might be lacking.

Why now?

There is a global wellbeing crisis, and it is affecting growing numbers of people all around the world. People are struggling for several reasons:

- **Lack of information** - they don't know how to change, what to do, or where to start.
- **Lack of resources** - they may have desire, but lack the necessary means to invest - information, technology, financially, time, place etc
- **Lack self-control** - they may have the information but they don't have the freedom and self-control to make positive changes. Life-limiting factors hinder their freedom.

Millions of people around the world are experiencing unfreedom, slaves to the desires that control them. The types of the desires that tend to ensnare people include video games, entertainment, gambling, drinking, smoking, drugs, pornography, caffeine or other stimulants, sports, or spending money. The list goes on.

These things affect people all over the world, from heads of state to those at the other end of society. Regardless of ethnicity, gender or age, people all across this vast globe are subject to this battle for freedom.

Why is the Human Bank different? The Soul

When it comes to wellness, everyone talks about our physical health, emotional health, relational health and mental health, but very few talk about the health of the soul. Our soul is our very core essence, our 'true self', comprised of our mind, will and emotions. Our thoughts, feelings, identity and desires all come from our soul.

So, if we leave our soul out of the wellbeing equation, we're leaving out the trunk of the tree and just trying to change the leaves. We cannot build true health and wellbeing if we neglect our soul. When our soul is damaged or in

5

poor health, we can experience a lack of peace, a lack of love, a lack of joy, a lack of energy, and a lack of freedom. This causes anxiety, fear, disconnection and loneliness, despair, hopelessness, and meaninglessness. We are like empty shells. With the right deposits, however, we can replenish peace, love, joy and energy.

Did you know there is a battle over your soul? This is because decision-making occurs in the soul. There is an enemy that seeks to steal your wellbeing through destructive investments, which is why we need a saviour who enables us to positively invest in our soul, bringing life, peace and true prosperity.

The reason *Human Bank*™ is so comprehensive is because it includes focus on the soul and how to build health and wellbeing in it, specifically, through connection with God. No, matter where you are in life, there is real hope in God.

With that in mind, I invite you on a journey to explore the concept of the Human Bank, and most importantly, *your* Human Bank. I hope that reading this book will begin a journey of discovery and increasing your understanding of true wellbeing. May it provide you with new awareness, new tools, new strategies, new inspiration, and new truth that empowers you to make real change and positive investments in your Human Bank, so that you truly prosper.

Chapter 1: The Ocean of Life

Have you ever felt like you had no idea who you really were, what your passions were, or what to do with your life?

A person with no clear purpose is like a boat floating on the ocean of life. Without a destination (purpose), or the motor, sail or oars (resources, time, health, connections, etc.) needed to get there, the boat will simply drift, not going anywhere in particular, at the mercy of the wind and the currents. It will end up wherever these external circumstances push them. Existence was the only purpose.

Or perhaps you feel like life is like a race, and you're sprinting to keep up. Consider these questions:

- Have you ever woken up and thought, *oh no, not another day*, struggling to get out of bed and open your eyes?
- Have you ever felt so tired and drained that it seemed as if the life and energy had been sucked right out of you?
- Have you ever felt as though your joy and happiness were left somewhere and you can't find them again?
- Have you ever felt without love? Disconnected, lonely, or without a sense of belonging?
- Have you ever felt so much confusion or anxiety that instead of peace, it felt like your heart was pounding and your head spinning?
- Have you ever had trouble focusing; maybe you go to work and stare at your computer screen trying to remember what you should be doing?
- Has there been a time when you wanted to do something so much that it occupied your thoughts constantly and you just had to do it?
- Have you ever felt like you lost your freedom to a life controlling habit?
- Have you ever been obsessed with something, or addicted to something that seemed to consume all your time, energy, money or focus? Where it feels like the addiction is the master and you're the servant?
- Ever felt like you lost your self-control and your freedom to decide?

Some of those may seem extreme, but they are common experiences for millions of people around the world. When we experience slavery to addictions, it is a sign our soul is in unfreedom. The good news is, you are not alone and there is hope!

Energy, joy, love, peace and freedom are fundamental needs for every human. In fact, they make up our Human Bank currency, which we must transact every day:

- **Energy** to empower our body's physical activity.
- **Joy** to empower our emotions.
- **Love,** whose experience allows us to have healthy interactions with other people, and ourselves.
- **Peace** to govern our minds.
- **Freedom** to empower our choice.

This is how they fall into the following Human Banks:

- Physical Bank - **Energy**
- Emotional Bank - **Joy**
- Relational Bank - **Love**
- Mental Bank - **Peace**
- Soul Bank - **Freedom**

People experiencing a deficit in any of these areas may not be able to cope with physical demands, process emotional pain, manage mental load, or resolve relational conflict (and often cause it).

When we do not have adequate quantities of Energy, Joy, Love, Peace and Freedom; our Human Bank is low, empty, or perhaps bankrupt. Life is a shadow of what we were designed to live. Like a car without fuel, we will not be able to make the journey.

Life is not a 100-metre sprint; it is a decades-long marathon. As such, we need to run at a pace that is sustainable for that time if we are to finish the race well. Too many people treat life like a sprint by running as fast as they can. Unfortunately, burnout can bring them to a halt before they reach the finish line. There are ways to know how to run the race well, so that is sustainable, beneficial and profitable to our wellbeing.

Let's begin that journey together. Let's explore the ocean of life and all its possibilities. First, we will focus on the two entities present in Human Bank.

The Human, and the Bank! We will define them and then how they merge to form the Human Bank.

First Part: The Human

What it is to be Human? Here are some definitions:

1. Biological Definition

Human (*Homo sapiens*): A species of bipedal primates belonging to the family Hominidae, distinguished by high cognitive abilities, complex language, and social structures.

2. Philosophical Definition

Human: A rational, self-aware being capable of abstract thought, morality, and self-determination. Often defined as a "thinking being" (res cogitans).

3. Theological Definition

Human: A creation made in the image of God (Imago Dei), possessing a soul and moral responsibility.

4. Psychological Definition

Human: A social, emotional, and cognitive being with consciousness, free will, and the ability to experience and interpret emotions.

5. Sociological Definition

Human: A member of a structured society, defined by culture, traditions, and interactions within groups and institutions. [1]

1: For Definition References, please see the footnote section (end of the book).

Given the earlier emphasis on the importance of soul wellbeing, I will focus on the spiritual aspect and elaborate on definition three, the theological definition:

> "Thus says God, the Lord, who created the heavens and stretched them out, who spread out the earth and what comes from it, who gives breath to the people on it and spirit to those who walk in it:" Isaiah 42:5

This passage clearly states that humans are more than animals; we are formed by and made for the living God, in His image, to know love, having an eternal soul, and specially created to be able to have a personal relationship with Him.

I understand that this may be an uncomfortable, even alien concept to some people, who may not wish to continue along this train of thought. However, I urge readers not to dismiss the notion based on preexisting thoughts and feelings or past hurts, upsets or experience. Allow me to discuss how foundational views of human existence affect our lives.

Firstly, if we are to know ourselves, we need to know where we originated, as that will add value and context to our present. The benefits that this can bring to your life includes love, meaning, joy and purpose. We are not the random result of a collision in the cosmos.

If we look at the Biblical narrative, one moment of creation stands out above all the rest. Each day of creation built upon the last, leading to the climax on the sixth day:

> "Then God said, 'Let us make man in our image, after our likeness. And let them have dominion over the fish of the sea and over the birds of the heavens and over the livestock and over all the earth and over every creeping thing that creeps on the earth.'" Genesis 1: 26.

What a remarkable statement for God to make about His greatest creations: us. It instantly elevates mankind above the rest of God's creation, for we were created in His image and likeness (that is, made to look like Him and to be like Him) and made to have dominion over it. Reproducing after one's image and likeness is an act of love, and reveals His heart for us.

Of course, the reproduction is not perfect, because Adam and Eve introduced sin into the world, and we are imperfect beings. The journey to knowing God as our Heavenly Father is such that as we draw closer to Him, we will see God reflected in our lives (in every area of wellbeing) more and more.

Sadly, too many people do not understand the uniqueness or significance of their creation, viewing themselves as, "just another human being", or worse a, random product of a meaningless big bang. Such thoughts are devaluing to you and I.

God didn't just want people created in His image; He wanted sons and daughters. He wanted a family that knew and loved their Father, who had a special relationship with Him. We can only imagine the joy God felt as He looked upon His new creation, with the same love and pride the most loving father looks upon a newborn child. We were designed to experience the love and enjoy the affection of our Heavenly Father.

Can you now see how special humankind is? For all of our flaws, we were designed by God Himself, to be His image and likeness on Earth. Genesis chapter 2 provides further details:

> "Then the Lord God formed the man of dust from the ground and breathed into his nostrils the breath of life, and the man became a living creature." Genesis 2:7

Here we see that the first human was formed from the dust of the earth, in the image of God. Then the Lord God breathed into this man (Adam) and he became a living creation, also like Him. The dust represents the physical aspect of a person's body, and the breath of God, the spirit that dwells within the body, giving it life. We are dualistic beings, comprised of a physical body and an eternal spirit.

This is amazing and distinguishes us from the rest of God's creation. We are chosen and created for a relationship with God.

Second Part: The Bank

We have examined the Human aspect of the Human Bank, understanding that we are uniquely created by God in His image and likeness, and this gives us intrinsic value, worth and meaning. The second concept is that of the Bank, so in this section let's look at what a banking system is.

The Banking System

Today, there are places of exchange where individuals and businesses can deposit money, withdraw money, borrow money or repay it. You're familiar with them: they're called banks. They help facilitate the way money is exchanged, through regulations designed to protect peoples' deposits and the bank's viability. For the purpose of this book, the simplest definition of a bank is a place in which we can deposit our money for safe storage, then withdraw from it, money when needed.

The Human Bank concept is based on the understanding that we make withdrawals from our Human Bank every day, but also encourages us to consider if we are also *depositing* into our Human Bank. If not, will we have resources/funds to draw on?

Bank Regulation and Financial Crisis

Regulation is crucial for any banking system. Governments regulate monetary policy so the banks fulfil their function for the community and the nation, which is to provide a stable financial system that people can access, utilise and benefit from.

One way that governments do this is by imposing what is called a "Loan to Debt Ratio" (LDR) which determines how much money banks can lend of the money that is deposited in them. For example, if the LDR is 50% and the bank has $100 deposited, then it can only lend out $50.

To put it simply banks cannot lend out more than the money that's deposited, and they must keep reserves if customers want to withdraw their money.

Money goes in and out of the bank in two ways: withdrawals and lending. Money goes into banks in two ways as well: through deposits and repayments of borrowed (loaned) money. The bank must have adequate money to service both individual withdrawals and the money that is lent out.

If banks do not maintain these ratios and do not have adequate money for customers to withdraw their money, then the bank is in default and insolvency regulators will step in to mitigate the financial situation and potentially shut it down. This has happened in the past, famously during the Global Financial Crisis of 2008. Banks lent above the safe lending ratios; not only that, but they onsold those loans to investors. Customers were most likely unaware of this practice. The loans originated from deposits by bank customers: individuals, families, businesses. They trusted the banks to keep their money safe for when they wanted to withdraw and access it.

The US housing market was booming. Loan assessment criteria were eased to the point of loans being approved for people who reportedly were without the ability to repay, including people who had no employment and previous poor repayment histories.

Mortgages were onsold to investors so the market was booming. People were buying homes, and everyone was happy. Then, suddenly in mid-2007 the housing market in the US started to decline and prices fell; the real estate bubble burst. People became increasingly unable to meet their repayments, defaults increased and over-inflated house prices came tumbling down. The assets devalued but the loans remained.

This created a ripple effect of local, then global panic as people pulled their money and investments out of banks, in effect withdrawing that money from the global monetary cycle. The circulation and exchange of money worldwide decreased. The rotation of the financial world slowed to a snail's pace.

The result was that prices dropped. The market started to correct itself; house prices fell but loan amounts remained high above their actual value. For example, people had taken out loans for five hundred thousand dollars on homes that were now valued at two hundred thousand dollars, leading to foreclosures. Dozens of banks closed in the United States, and globally. They were insolvent primarily due to excessive lending to people who didn't have the capacity to repay. When these people defaulted on their loan repayments, banks defaulted on their own repayments and the cycle went down the line, affecting financial institutions and businesses worldwide. It became known as the "Global Financial Crisis" (GFC) or "2008 financial crisis".

The Global Financial Crisis of 2008 is in some ways a mirror of the Global Wellbeing Crisis that we find ourselves in today. The wellbeing crisis comes about when we spend all our wellbeing currency and do not have enough left for our daily withdrawals (i.e. the demands or work and life). We are in deficit, unable to meet our daily wellbeing demands. Do you feel like one or more parts of your Human Bank are bankrupt with nothing left to withdraw? If so, what are the impacts? We will explore this as we progress in the book.

Chapter 2: The Wellbeing Crisis

If a plant goes without water or fertiliser, it cannot thrive. Starved of its essential nutrients, it may become stunted instead of reaching its full potential. Humans are the same way. When we are deprived of energy, joy, love, peace and freedom, we do not achieve our full potential or productivity, which negatively affects our quality of life. There are two factors which could cause this deficit:

1. We withdraw more from our Human Bank than we deposit.

2. We make negative investments into our Human Bank.

The problem is that most of our lifestyles impact us negatively in some way. We deprive body and soul of what they need to thrive. This has created a crisis of wellbeing, felt by people all across the globe. Below are some statistics that highlight the challenges people face.

Communicable Diseases are diseases that are infectious and are transmitted from one person to another. **Noncommunicable Diseases (NCDs) are not spread, they are developed.** Tackling the rapidly growing global burden of NCDs constitutes one of the major challenges for development in the 21st century. During the first two decades of the century, global deaths due to NCDs and mental health rapidly increased (Fig. 1).

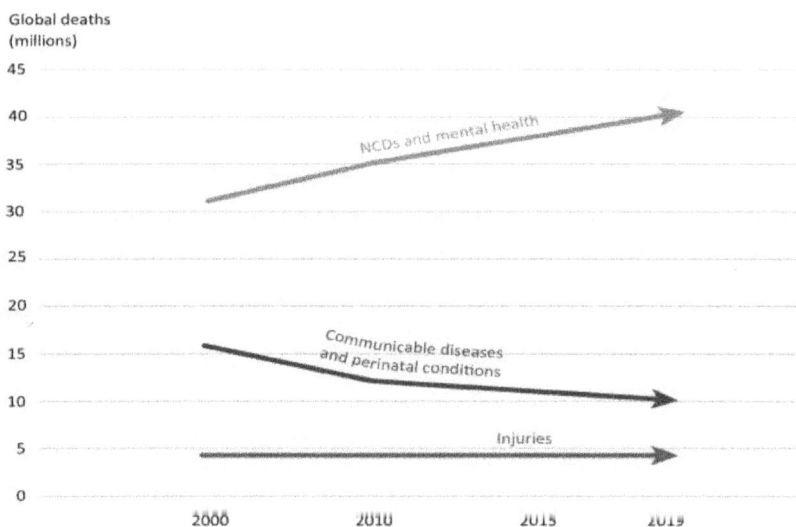

Global deaths (millions)

NCDs and mental health

Communicable diseases and perinatal conditions

Injuries

2000   2010   2015   2019

FIG. 1. Increase in global deaths due to NCDs and mental health (2000-2019)2

The global share of NCD deaths among all deaths increased from 61% in 2000 to 74% in 2019.This is a significant change. Note that this was not an overall increase in human population, but an increase in the overall percentage of deaths caused by noncommunicable diseases. It is shocking that 74% of all deaths globally are caused by noncommunicable diseases, which are often preventable.

What does this tell us? That increasing amounts of people are dying due to *preventable* diseases such as heart issues, cancer, diabetes, respiratory diseases, and mental health issues with an increase of 13% in nineteen years from 2000-2019. We have to change this!

FIG. 2. Deaths from NCDs by age group.

NCD deaths (age)	2000 (millions)	2010 (millions)	2015 (millions)	2019 (millions)
>70 years	16.8	19.9	21.8	23.8
30-70 years	12.7	13.7	14.7	15.7
<30 years	1.7	1.5	1.4	1.4
Total deaths	31.2	35.1	37.9	40.9

3

FIG. 3. Deaths from NCD's in those aged 30-70 years

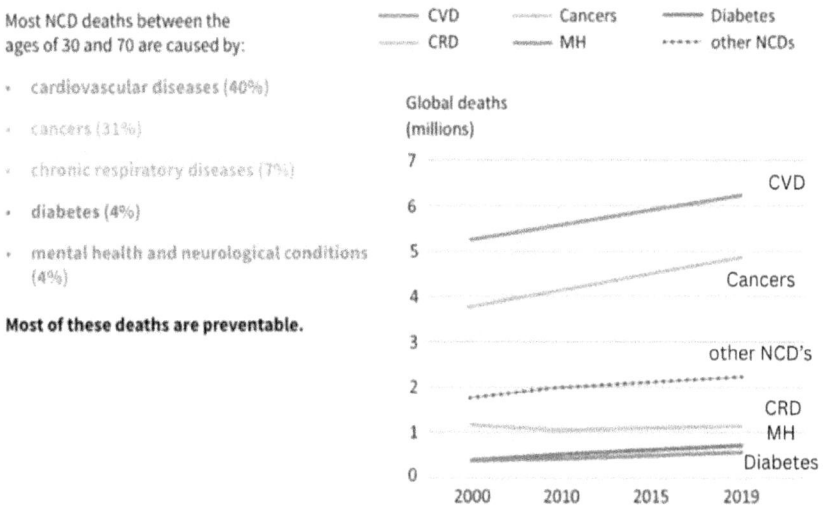

Most NCD deaths between the ages of 30 and 70 are caused by:

- cardiovascular diseases (40%)
- cancers (31%)
- chronic respiratory diseases (7%)
- diabetes (4%)
- mental health and neurological conditions (4%)

Most of these deaths are preventable.

4

Most NCD deaths between the ages of 30 and 70 are caused by:

- cardiovascular diseases (40%)

- cancers (31%)

- chronic respiratory diseases (7%)

- diabetes (4%)

- mental health and neurological conditions (4%)

People are at their most economically productive between the ages of 30 and 70, and the death of people in this age group caused by NCDs (considered "premature deaths") is rapidly increasing.

Why is that? There are several key factors which affect life expectancy and can contribute to premature death:

1. Genetics – Family history and hereditary diseases.

2. Healthcare Access – Availability of medical services and treatments.

3. Lifestyle Choices – Diet, exercise, smoking, and alcohol consumption.

4. Economic Status – Wealth and access to resources.

5. Environmental Factors – Pollution, climate, and living conditions.

6. Public Health Policies – Vaccination programs, disease control, and sanitation.

There are of course factors outside of the control of the individual which nevertheless can impact their life expectancy, including genetics, healthcare access, environmental factors and public health policies. However, notice that lifestyle choices is one of the causes of NCD deaths. That is exactly what they are: choices we make about how to live. Consider the fact that many deaths could be preventable by modifying lifestyle. For this reason, we will focus on why your lifestyle choices are important and how they have a significant impact on your overall health and wellbeing, quality of life and life expectancy.

Causes of Non-Communicable Diseases (NCDs)

Non-communicable diseases (NCDs) are chronic medical conditions. They often develop due to a combination of genetic, environmental, and lifestyle factors. Let's explore some of those major causes of non-communicable diseases in more detail:

1. **Unhealthy Diet**

    - High consumption of processed foods, sugar, salt, and unhealthy fats.
    - Leads to obesity, diabetes, cardiovascular diseases, and hypertension.

2. **Physical Inactivity**

    - Lack of exercise contributes to heart disease, stroke, obesity, and type 2 diabetes.

3. **Tobacco Use**

    - Causes lung cancer, chronic respiratory diseases, cardiovascular diseases, and stroke.

4. **Excessive Alcohol Consumption**

    - Increases risk of liver diseases, high blood pressure, heart disease, and certain cancers.

5. **Genetic & Hereditary Factors**

    - Some NCDs, like diabetes, cancer, and heart disease, have a genetic predisposition.
    - Family history plays a role but can be managed with lifestyle changes.

6. **Environmental Factors**

    - Air pollution contributes to respiratory diseases (asthma, lung cancer).
    - Exposure to harmful chemicals increases the risk of chronic illnesses.

7. **Aging**

- Aging naturally increases the risk of conditions like Alzheimer's, osteoporosis, and cardiovascular diseases.

8. **Stress & Mental Health Disorders**

- Chronic stress, anxiety, and depression can lead to heart disease, high blood pressure, and weakened immunity.[5]

Common Non-Communicable Diseases:

1. **Cardiovascular Diseases** (Heart attacks, strokes, hypertension)

2. **Cancer** (Lung, breast, prostate, colorectal)

3. **Chronic Respiratory Diseases** (Asthma, chronic obstructive pulmonary disease - COPD)

4. **Diabetes** (Type 1 & Type 2)

5. **Neurological Disorders** (Alzheimer's, Parkinson's disease)

6. **Kidney and Liver Diseases** (chronic kidney disease, cirrhosis) [6]

Facts & Statistics

World Health Organization (WHO):

- NCDs account for 74% of all global deaths (41 million people annually).
- Cardiovascular diseases are the leading cause, responsible for 17.9 million deaths per year.
- Diabetes has quadrupled in prevalence since 1980.
- Lung diseases, often caused by smoking and pollution, kill over 4 million people annually. [7]

Centres for Disease Control and Prevention (CDC):

- 6 out of 10 adults in the U.S. have an NCD.
- 4 out of 10 have **two or more** chronic diseases.

- NCDs cost the U.S. healthcare system **$3.8 trillion annually**. 8

The table below uses this data to emphasise the connection between risk factors and chronic disease.

Evidence and connection of Risk Factors and Chronic Disease

Cause of NCD	Kidney & Liver Diseases	Chronic Respiratory Diseases	Cardio-vascular Diseases	Neuro-logical Disorders	Diabetes	Cancer
Unhealthy Diet	7	4	9	5	10	6
Physical Inactivity	5	3	8	4	9	5
Tobacco Use	6	10	7	2	3	9
Excessive Alcohol	10	5	6	3	4	7
Stress & Mental Health	5	6	7	7	6	5

9

These five risk factors increase the likelihood of developing one of the major chronic diseases which can lead to premature death as we can see in the table on the following page.

Non-Communicable Diseases – Common Symptoms and Lifestyle Impacts

Non-Communicable Disease	Common Symptoms	Lifestyle Impact
Cardiovascular Diseases	Chest pain, shortness of breath, irregular heartbeat, fatigue	Limited physical activity, dietary restrictions, medication dependence

Cancer	Unexplained weight loss, persistent pain, abnormal lumps, fatigue	Physical and emotional toll, dietary adjustments, treatment side effects
Chronic Respiratory Diseases	Chronic cough, wheezing, shortness of breath, chest tightness	Reduced lung function, dependency on inhalers, environmental sensitivity
Diabetes	Frequent urination, excessive thirst, fatigue, blurred vision	Dietary restrictions, insulin or medication dependency, risk of complications
Neurological Disorders	Memory loss, difficulty speaking, muscle tremors, confusion	Cognitive decline, loss of independence, emotional and social impact
Kidney & Liver Diseases	Swelling, fatigue, loss of appetite, nausea, yellowing of skin	Dietary restrictions, fluid intake control, frequent medical visits

Note: For evidence and references, see the *Footnotes* section.

The WHO indicates that these non-communicable diseases are caused by risk factors and lifestyle factors, and modifiable risk behaviours:

> "Well-established evidence shows that the incidence of cancer, cardiovascular disease, chronic respiratory disease and diabetes share modifiable risk factors such as alcohol consumption, body mass index (BMI), cigarette smoking, unhealthy diet and physical inactivity, which account for more than two-thirds of these diseases."[10]

Yes, there can be biological, genetic, environmental or other factors, but we are specifically focusing on behavioural and lifestyle factors that contribute to these diseases. In other words, things that we can do that decrease our risk of developing these diseases.

Optimal physical wellbeing requires good health and vitality. Our bodies are designed in such a way that they need certain things to thrive. If we substitute those things for alternatives, for example, filling up on soft drink or alcohol instead of drinking water, we deprive our bodies of the things that it actually needs to function well. There are many substances and chemicals that can be found in foods and drinks that can be detrimental to our physical health, particularly when consumed in large quantities. Things like alcohol, unnatural manufactured and processed drinks and food high in artificial chemicals, salts and sugars. At best it is like putting a very poor grade of petrol into the fuel tank of the car; at worst it is causing damage to the engine that could even prevent the vehicle from operating.

Without optimal fuel (good nutrition), our engine (body) will not be able to operate at peak efficiency. This results in us becoming lethargic, easily tired, burnt out, or worse. If we try to fuel our bodies on foods and drinks that are deficient in nutrients or downright harmful, it potentially could lead to developing one (or more) of the diseases referred to above.

What about the other areas of wellbeing: emotional, mental, relational and soulful? What impact does our physical wellbeing have on these? Poor physical health can contribute to emotional, mental and relational issues such as tiredness, anxiety, depression, irritability, difficulty concentrating and frustration.

Clearly there are investments we can make into our Human Bank which are harmful to our wellbeing. Fortunately, there are also many positive things we can deposit into it, so that we when we have a physical, emotional, relational, mental or soulful need, what we withdraw from our bank is also positive.

We have seen the major risk factors that can contribute to chronic diseases, and have considered how many of them can be managed, through behaviour modification, to reduce or prevent risk. Some factors are beyond our control; however, others are within our power to change. What we invest into our bodies is our choice, and will determine whether the return on our investment is positive or negative. This is really what the Human Bank is all about. It's about our positive and negative investments which can either produce a positive return or a negative return. The purpose of this book is to increase awareness of the positive investments we can make into our physical, emotional, relational, mental and soul banks to achieve total wellbeing.

The focus of this book is things that are within our control. We are not just victims of circumstance, without hope. We are empowered by choice; your choices can result in vitality and wellbeing. There is hope in God, and we can make real change in our lives. Consider Matthew 19:26: "But Jesus looked at them and said, 'With man this is impossible, but with God all things are possible.'"

Of course, there are factors in our life that may dominate us and lead us into destructive behaviours that harm our wellbeing, but *Human Bank* addresses the negative investments we make as well as the positive ones we should choose. Why do we indulge in destructive behaviours that we know can hurt us? Even knowing that they can cause disease and or lead to premature death? There are plenty of well-known examples:

- Cigarette packaging comes with a warning that smoking kills, yet some people keep smoking.
- Driving under the influence of alcohol is dangerous, but people still risk their own lives, and others' on the road.
- Drugs can alter the chemistry of our brain and our way of thinking, often permanently, but people still take them.
- Excessive alcohol consumption can cause liver disease and damage the brain, yet some people drink all their lives.
- Gambling can be addictive, but some people still risk large amounts of money in it.
- Pornography is destructive, yet some people choose to indulge in it rather than have real, healthy relationships.
- Excessive screen time can be distracting and time-consuming, yet we can't seem to put down the tablet or turn off the television.

The list goes on. As a society we have generally been educated on these risk factors, and have awareness of the importance of reducing them. So why do we continue indulging in self-destructive behaviours that go against self-preservation, even to the point that they can cause diseases and premature death? Because they're addictive. The argument I put forward here is that there is a better way to live and addictions can be broken so that we experience wellbeing in every area.

Let's explore the possibilities so that collectively we can improve our quality of life and lifespan, having healthier and more meaningful lives for the betterment of not only ourselves, but also for our partners, families, friends, workplaces, communities and nations.

Chapter 3: The Human Bank™

In the previous chapters we examined the concepts of Human, Bank, and looked at the global wellbeing crisis and how most major noncommunicable diseases are often preventable and caused predominantly by four risk factors. Now, let's look at our Human Bank.

We are familiar with the banking concept and the role banks play in helping us to manage our money, and how we make transactions by withdrawing and depositing currency. Then there is also how we spend our money and the motivations behind those transactions. What do those purchases give us? What physical, emotional or other benefits do we get in return for our money? They could vary based on our needs, desires.

We have varying levels of understanding of our whole-life wellbeing. General public knowledge informs us that we need to be healthy; exercise, perhaps get regular medical check-ups and be aware of what might be harmful to our health. The purpose of this chapter is to broaden our awareness and understanding of whole-life wellbeing by examining the five Human Bank areas. This is so that we are well equipped to manage and invest in our whole-life wellbeing, in turn enabling us to really flourish and prosper.

Defining Human Bank™:

"Human Bank™ represents our whole-life wellbeing. By integrating economic theory with ancient Biblical truths, it empowers us to assess, measure, and invest in our wellbeing, enabling us to truly prosper in both our soul and our Human Bank."

Founder – Michael J. Smith

How does economic theory and biblical truth combine into a wellbeing framework? That is something that we will explore and unpack together throughout this book. People may be wondering, how could there be any correlation between the two? They are not contradictory because they both enable us to assess our overall wellbeing and the reasons behind our decisions. Let's unpack this a bit further. But for now, the key takeaway is that your Human Bank represents your overall life wellbeing. Whole-life wellbeing involves incorporating our physical, emotional, relational, mental and soul areas of life. These wellbeing areas were first discussed in the introduction, and are our five Human Banks:

- **Physical Human Bank™**

- **Emotional Human Bank™**

- **Relational Human Bank™**

- **Mental Human Bank™**

- **Soul Human Bank™**

The Human Bank is a holistic concept that represents our overall wellbeing across multiple domains—physical, emotional, relational, mental, and soul. It involves the positive or negative transactions of various forms of 'currency', such as: joy, energy, love, peace, and freedom. These transactions either contribute to a profit (feeling fulfilled, balanced, and healthy) or a loss (feeling drained, stressed, or disconnected), ultimately influencing our overall sense of wellbeing.

Why a bank, you may ask? The bank analogy helps us to understand that we have different currencies that we transact every day in different areas of our lives. It also encourages us to consider whether we are experiencing a loss or deficit in any area, and whether we have the resources to profit in each area of our Human Bank. Overall, it provides a good framework to help conceptualise, quantify, assess, measure, and invest in a whole-life wellbeing.

We will now explore the concept in detail, including ways that we can invest into the different areas of our Human Bank and the returns on our investments. Here is a summary of each bank and the currency it uses:

- The **Physical Human Bank** represents our overall physical wellbeing and the transaction of **energy** in our daily lives. This results in our Physical Bank being in profit (feeling energised and healthy) or in loss (feeling fatigued or depleted).

- The **Emotional Human Bank** represents our overall emotional wellbeing and the transactions of its currency, **joy**, in our daily lives. This results in our Emotional Bank being in profit (feeling emotionally fulfilled) or in loss (feeling emotionally drained).
- The **Relational Human Bank** represents our overall relational wellbeing and the transactions of our **love** currency. This results in our Relational Bank being profitable (relationships thriving) or in loss (relationships struggling).
- The **Mental Human Bank** represents our overall mental wellbeing and the transactions of **peace** in our daily lives. This results in our Mental Bank being in profit (feeling mentally at peace) or in loss (feeling stressed or overwhelmed).
- The **Soul Human Bank** represents our overall soul wellbeing and the transaction of the currency **freedom** in our daily lives. This results in our Soul Bank being in profit (feeling fulfilled and aligned with purpose) or in loss (feeling restricted or disconnected).

Human Bank™ Concept

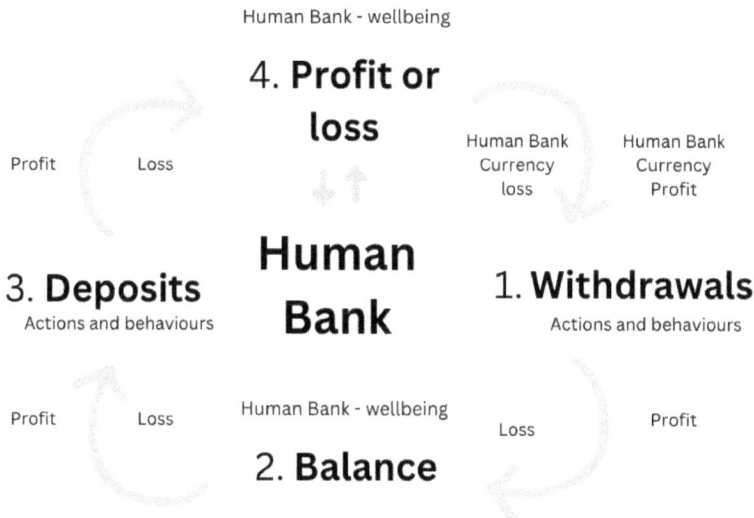

Human Bank - wellbeing

4. Profit or loss

Profit   Loss

Human Bank Currency loss   Human Bank Currency Profit

Human Bank

3. Deposits
Actions and behaviours

1. Withdrawals
Actions and behaviours

Profit   Loss

Human Bank - wellbeing

Loss   Profit

2. Balance

In the coming chapters we will explore further:

- What are our daily withdrawals and how do they impact our Human Bank?

- What influences our investments into our Human Bank

- What are the deposits that we make into our Human Bank and how do they translate to profit or loss?

- What *is* profit and loss in the Human Bank?

All four of these aspects of the Human Bank we will cover in depth so that you can have a solid understanding of the Human Bank, how it works, and how it applies to your life so that you can invest for true profit. For now, let's look at the five Human Banks.

1. The Physical Human Bank™

Physical wellbeing

Definition: Physical wellbeing refers to the state of the body's health, fitness, and functioning. It encompasses aspects like maintaining a balanced diet, regular physical activity, adequate sleep, and avoiding harmful habits like smoking or overconsumption of alcohol. This is also about the ability to perform daily activities without discomfort or restrictions. 11

Physical Human Bank

Definition: Represents our overall physical wellbeing and the transactions of our energy currency resources in our daily lives. This results in our Physical Bank being in profit (feeling energised and healthy) or in loss (feeling fatigued or depleted).

Introduction: The Physical Bank represents the state of our physical health and energy resources.

Currency: The currency in the Physical Bank is **Energy**.

- **Deposits:** We deposit Energy through healthy habits such as exercise, sleep, and proper nutrition.

- **Withdrawals:** We withdraw Energy through stress, illness, poor diet, and lack of rest.

Profit Indicators: Having abundant Energy for the daily withdrawals of life and to help others.

- Feeling energised, healthy, and strong; improved stamina; better sleep quality.

Loss Indicators: Not having abundant Energy for the daily withdrawals of life and to help others.

- Chronic fatigue, poor health, illness, sleep deprivation.

Investment Strategies: Regular physical activity, healthy eating, enough sleep, stress management practices.

Investment Actions:

1. Daily, I eat a healthy and nutritious diet (high in fruit & vegetables and low in fat, salt, sugar).

2. Daily, I engage in 30–60 minutes of exercise.

3. Daily, I exercise self-control to avoid unhealthy coping mechanisms (e.g., excessive eating, excessive drinking, avoidance, substance use, isolation, excessive screen time, media, or shopping) to deal with stress, anxiety, or negative emotions.

Conclusion: Prioritising physical health leads to higher energy levels, better immunity, greater overall vitality and reduced risk of major chronic diseases.

2. The Emotional Human Bank™

Emotional Wellbeing

Definition: Emotional wellbeing involves the ability to recognise, understand, express, and manage one's emotions in a healthy way. It's about having a positive outlook, emotional balance, and the resilience to cope with stress, life challenges, and setbacks while nurturing self-acceptance and self-compassion.
12

Emotional Human Bank

Definition: Represents our overall emotional wellbeing and the transactions of our joy currency in our daily lives. This results in our Emotional Bank being in profit (feeling emotionally fulfilled) or in loss (feeling emotionally drained).

Introduction: The Emotional Bank represents our emotional health and wellbeing.

Currency: The currency in the Emotional Bank is **Joy.**

- **Deposits:** We deposit Joy by living in accordance with our 'true self'; that is, our values and purpose, processing emotional hurts and expressing gratitude.

- **Withdrawals:** We withdraw Joy by not living in alignment with our 'true self', our values and purpose, and by not processing emotional hurts and not expressing gratitude.

Profit Indicators: Having abundant joy for the daily withdrawals of life and to encourage others.

- Feeling joyful, emotionally balanced, happy, and resilient; strong emotional intelligence and fulfillment.

Loss Indicators: Not having abundant joy for the daily withdrawals of life and or encourage others.

- Feeling drained, overwhelmed, anxious, or emotionally down and disconnected.

Investment Strategies: Practicing gratitude, spending time helping others, living your 'True self', managing stress, expressing emotions healthily.

Investment Actions:

1. Each day, heal emotional upset by processing feelings, releasing anger, and letting go of bitterness and resentment.

2. Each day, live in alignment with my authentic 'true self'; my values, beliefs, passions, and purpose.

3. Each day, express gratitude, recognising that while I may not have everything I want or need, I am content with my life.

Conclusion: Investing in emotional health increases our ability to live in alignment with our true self, values, and purpose, empowering us to live a life of meaning and fulfilment. Processing hurts and upsets frees us from the past and releases us into our future and healthier relationships.

3. The Relational Human Bank™

Relational Wellbeing

Definition: Relational wellbeing refers to the quality of one's interpersonal relationships. It includes positive, supportive, and healthy interactions with family, friends, and the wider community. Key elements include trust, empathy, communication, and the feeling of social connectedness. [13]

Relational Human Bank

Definition: Represents our overall relational health and the transactions of our love currency in our daily lives. This results in our Relational Bank being in profit (relationships thriving) or in loss (relationships struggling).

Introduction: The Relational Human bank relates to the quality, connection and health of our relationships with ourselves and others.

Currency: The currency in the Relational Bank is **Love**.

- **Deposits:** We deposit Love by supporting and loving others, cultivating authentic selfless relationships and not for gain.

- **Withdrawals:** You withdraw Love by not supporting and loving others, not cultivating authentic relationships and loving money or things more than people.

Deposits: We deposit Love by supporting and loving others, cultivating authentic relationships and not loving money or things.

Withdrawals: You withdraw Love by not supporting and loving others, not cultivating authentic relationships and loving money.

Profit Indicators: Having abundant Love for the daily withdrawals of life and to love others.

- Strong connections, loved and loving others, healthy self-worth, identity and thriving relationships.

Loss Indicators: Not having abundant Love for the daily withdrawals of life and to love others.

- Lack of love, loneliness, communication breakdowns, conflict, and isolation.

Investment Strategies: Active listening, serving and supporting others, expressing gratitude, spending quality time, resolving conflicts respectfully, financial wellbeing.

Investment Actions:

1. Each day, I offer help and support to those in need in my life.

2. Each day, I cultivate deep, authentic relationships with people who uplift and support me.

3. Each day, I have enough money for essentials and spend my money wisely, avoiding debt.

Conclusion: Investing in and guarding relationships creates deeper bonds, greater love, connection, mutual support, and a more fulfilling empowering life.

4. The Mental Human Bank™

Mental Wellbeing

Definition: Mental wellbeing refers to cognitive and psychological aspects of health, including mental clarity, focus, and emotional resilience. It involves the ability to cope with stress, solve problems, make decisions, and maintain a positive mental outlook on life. Mental wellbeing is integral to handling day-to-day challenges while maintaining a sense of self-worth and balance. 14

The Mental Bank

Definition: Represents our overall mental health and the transactions of our **peace** currency in our daily lives. This results in our Mental Bank being in profit (feeling peace and clarity of mind) or in loss (feeling stressed or overwhelmed).

Introduction: The Mental Bank represents our mental health and mind wellbeing.

Currency: The currency in the Mental Bank is **Peace**.

- **Deposits:** We deposit Peace through forgiving ourselves and others, living with a sense of meaning and purpose and trusting God.

- **Withdrawals:** We withdraw Peace through not forgiving ourselves and others, not living with a sense of meaning and purpose or not trusting God.

Peace is lost when we invest in negative media, cognitive overload, toxic thoughts, or holding onto bitterness and unforgiveness.

Profit Indicators: Having abundant Peace for the daily withdrawals of life and to give peace to others.

- Peace of mind, clear thinking, focus, calmness, mental clarity, reduced anxiety.

Loss Indicators: Not having abundant Peace for the daily withdrawals of life and or to give peace to others.

- Lack of peace of mind, overwhelm, stress, poor concentration, negative thinking patterns.

Investment Strategies: Trust God, live with meaning and purpose, practice forgiveness, practice being still in God.

Investment Actions:

1. Each day, I practice forgiveness— giving and receiving— for others and for myself.

2. Each day, I live with a sense of meaning and purpose that guides my actions.

3. Each day, I trust in God with things beyond my control.

Conclusion: We invest into our Mental Bank by forgiving ourselves and others, living with a sense of meaning and purpose and trusting God. This brings peace of mind, which leads to greater clarity, productivity, decision-making, and overall wellbeing.

5. Soul Human Bank™

Soul Wellbeing

Definition: Soul wellbeing relates to an individual's spiritual health and inner peace, often associated with a sense of purpose, meaning, and alignment with one's values. For some, it may be related to religious or spiritual beliefs, while for others, it may involve personal fulfillment, self-reflection, and a deep connection to their life's purpose.15

The Soul Bank

Definition: Represents our overall soul health and the transactions of the currency **Freedom** in our daily lives. This results in our Soul Bank being in profit (feeling free, fulfilled and aligned with purpose) or in loss (feeling restricted or disconnected).

Introduction: The Soul Bank represents our spiritual freedom and wellbeing.

Currency: The currency in the Soul Bank is **Freedom**. We deposit Freedom by living in alignment with our purpose and values.

- **Deposits:** You deposit Freedom by having faith in God, daily living to love God and others, maintaining daily personal prayer and Bible reading.

- **Withdrawals:** You withdraw Freedom by not having faith in God, not showing love to God and others daily, not maintaining daily personal prayer and personal Bible reading.

Profit Indicators: Having abundant Freedom for the daily withdrawals of life and to give Freedom to others.

- Connection with God, a deep sense of purpose, inner peace, spiritual fulfillment, alignment with values.

Loss Indicators: Not having abundant Freedom for the daily withdrawals of life nor giving Freedom to others.

- Separation from God. feelings of emptiness, lack of peace, meaning, hope, disconnection from self or spiritual beliefs.

Investment Strategies: Having faith in God, daily living to love God and others, maintaining daily personal prayer and Bible reading.

Investment Actions:

1. Each day, I experience a connection to my faith in God that brings me love, peace, and hope.

2. Each day, I live to love and honour God and others with my actions.

3. Each day, I dedicate time to prayer and personal reflection.

Conclusion: Invest in your soul through faith, living to love God and others and practicing daily habits of prayer. This will provide a deeper sense of love, peace, a greater love for and understanding of truth, meaning, and connectedness to God and others.

Chapter 4: The Human Bank™ Currency

Just like a financial bank, the Human Bank operates with different types of currencies, with each currency representing a core aspect of our Human Bank. Each currency can be deposited, withdrawn, or spent, influencing the overall profitability of our Human Bank. We need to know what we are depositing and withdrawing, so that we can measure it.

Human Bank™ Currency - Definition

The essential resource each of the Five Human Banks needs to operate and flourish. Human Bank™ Currency - Energy, Joy, Love, Peace, and Freedom is deposited through positive investments and withdrawn to meet daily demands. By investing through the 15 Human Bank™ Investments, individuals replenish their Banks to sustain wellbeing and capacity for life.

- Physical Human Bank™ - currency is **Energy**

- Emotional Human Bank™ - currency is **Joy**

- Relational Human Bank™ - currency is **Love**

- Mental Human Bank™ - currency is **Peace**

- Soul Human Bank™ - currency is **Freedom**

Thinking of these five aspects as currency enables us to follow the banking analogy of depositing or withdrawing. As we grow in awareness of our five Human Bank currencies, we also grow in awareness of how we can withdraw those currencies, and how we deposit them - this is the crucial role and function of the Human Bank.

We will look in greater detail at the investments we can make in the coming chapter. But for now, here is a brief overview of the topics we will look at regarding the currencies of the Human Bank:

- The concept of **Counterfeit Currency**; what we sometimes invest into our Human Banks, even though they are inferior substitutes for energy, joy, love, peace and freedom.

- The concept of **True Currency**. In other words, what we should really be investing in our Human Banks.

- An in-detail look at the currencies of the five Human Banks; what they are, how to deposit and withdraw them, and the counterfeits.

Counterfeit Currency

The government-endorsed, legal tender used for money in a certain country is that nation's national currency. However, sometimes counterfeit money circulates in a nation which looks suitable to use but actually it has no value and should not be used as currency.

Human Bank™ Counterfeit/Foreign Currency

What happens when we are in the state of loss/bankruptcy in our Human Bank Currency? We turn to alternative sources of supply called **Counterfeit Currency**.

For the purposes of the Human Bank, think of counterfeit currency as something that can be invested, but shouldn't be. It is an inferior substitute for the genuine human bank currencies of energy, joy, love peace or freedom. It can cause harm and result in profit loss, and should be exchanged for genuine Human Bank currency.

Later in this book, we actually assess these foreign currencies and some of their potential impacts. This is because they have a significant impact on our wellbeing. Yes, using a counterfeit currency may seem like a 'quick fix' but the long-term impacts on our life, wellbeing and our Human Bank are usually negative. We need to assess them and be aware of how we might be negatively investing foreign currency into our Human Banks, so that we can avoid them and invest in true Human Bank currency. The improvements to our quality of life is worth it in the long-term. There really is no adequate substitute for energy, joy, love, peace and freedom. Let's look at the currencies of the five Human Banks in further detail.

It is critical to understand what the five Human Bank Currencies are so that we recognise the counterfeits as inferior substitutes. Before we examine these in more detail, there is another currency I would like to introduce.

True Currency

What is True Currency? And how do we receive it? True Currency is the most significant and valuable currency of the Human Banks as it produces exponential life, energy, joy, love, peace, and freedom. Think of it as the ultimate currency!

There are investments that we make to produce Human Bank Currency, and another investment which produces True Currency. This currency is a spiritual currency that is produced by faith and relationship with God. It is the thing that produces true life, true energy, true joy, true peace, and true love in their purest, most fulfilling forms. With this True Currency, our souls truly prosper.

We will explore this further on.

The Five Human Banks and Their Currencies

How can we profitably invest in our five Human Banks? Here is a detailed look at the currencies we use.

Physical Human Bank™ Currency: Energy

Deposits: We deposit **Energy** through healthy habits such as exercise, sleep, and proper nutrition.

Withdrawals: We withdraw **Energy** through unhealthy habits such as lack of exercise, sleep, and proper nutrition.

Counterfeit Currency: Artificial Sources; energy stimulants such as caffeine and other drinks provide temporary boosts.

True Currency: Energy; true spiritual Energy comes from God. It helps us develop self-control through a healthy soul; inner discipline enables us to make positive physical investments.

Spending Energy: Work and life responsibilities, excessive demands, unhealthy behaviours, and obligations deplete energy.

Emotional Human Bank™ Currency: Joy

Deposits: We deposit **Joy** by living in alignment with our 'true self' (i.e. our values and purpose, processing emotional hurts and expressing gratitude), and by engaging in meaningful and fulfilling activities such as supporting others, self-care, hobbies, and other positive interactions – making a difference.

Withdrawals: We withdraw **Joy** by not living in alignment with our 'true self'; that is, in accordance to our values and purpose, by not processing emotional hurts and not expressing gratitude.

Counterfeit Currency: Media and entertainment; temporary experiences we seek to bring happiness but do not provide joy or fulfillment.

True Currency: Joy; comes from a connection with God; a spiritual relationship with God prevents depletion and overflows into our life.

Spending Joy: Given away to stress, negativity, and unwanted obligations—things we "have to do" that drain emotional wellbeing.

♡ Relational Human Bank™ Currency: Love

Deposits: We deposit **Love** by supporting and loving others, cultivating authentic relationships and not loving money and possessions. Specifically,

giving love through meaningful relationships, selflessness, and acts of love and service.

Withdrawals: You withdraw **Love** through selfishness; by not supporting and loving others, not cultivating authentic relationships and loving money. Love is taken away by selfishness, self-centredness, withholding love or keeping love for ourselves, unforgiveness, and destructive relationships.

Counterfeit Currency: Pornography; love gets misdirected into selfishness, self-satisfaction, or unhealthy desires rather than selfless love.

True Currency: Love; being loved through a relationship with God fills our relational bank with unconditional love, enabling us to love both God and others.

Spending Love: It can be given to self or others, but it can also be withheld, distorted, or spent on the wrong priorities.

Mental Human Bank™ Currency: Peace

Deposits: We deposit **Peace** through forgiving ourselves and others, living with a sense of meaning and purpose and trusting God.

Withdrawals: We withdraw **Peace** through not forgiving ourselves and others, not living with a sense of meaning and purpose or not trusting God. **Peace** is lost when we invest in negative media, toxic thoughts, or hold onto unforgiveness.

Counterfeit Currency: Substance use; using substances to compensate for a lack of peace. Anxiety, worry, mental oppression, and unfulfilled desires steal peace.

True Currency: Peace; trusting in God overcomes anxiety and fear, granting us deep inner peace.

Spending Peace: Worrying about things beyond our control, consuming negative media, cognitive overload and engaging in unresolved conflicts.

Soul Human Bank™ Currency: Freedom

Deposits: You deposit **Freedom** by having faith in God, daily living to love God and others, maintaining daily personal prayer and personal Bible reading. Freedom is gained by living in alignment with our purpose, trusting in and surrendering to God, and walking in truth.

Withdrawals: You withdraw **Freedom** by not having faith in God, not daily living to love God and others, not maintaining daily personal prayer and personal Bible reading. Freedom is lost to addictions, being a slave to pleasure, materialism, debt and unhealthy dependencies.

Counterfeit Currency: Addiction; spiritual bondage and loss of autonomy weakens your sense of freedom.

True Currency: Freedom; true freedom comes from a spiritual connection with God, bringing light to our soul and freeing us from darkness and evil.

Spending Freedom: Giving it away to screens, substances, gambling, porn, drinking, drugs, sex, escapism, and worldly distractions etc.

Summary

Managing the Human Bank requires intentionality: intentional deposits, mindful, guarded withdrawals, and wise spending of our Human Bank currency to maintain overall wellbeing.

By investing in our Human Bank, we can avoid the need for counterfeit currency, and we build a life of energy, joy, love, peace, and freedom in God.

Chapter 5: The Human Bank™ Investments

Investments are incredibly important. They either produce a return (profit), or a loss. It is the same with our investments in wellbeing through Human Banks.

Human Bank™ Investments - Definition

Human Bank™ Investments are the 15 Positive and 15 Negative evidence-based wellbeing actions that either contribute to or deplete the five Human Banks - Physical, Emotional, Relational, Mental, and Soul.

Key Human Bank Principles:

- If we make a positive investment we will get a profitable return on our investment.
- If we make a negative investment we will get a negative return on our investment.

Let's look at the positive and negative investments that we can make and how they impact our five Human Banks.

The following 15 Positive Investments and 15 and Negative Investments are carefully selected, evidence-based wellbeing factors which either positively or negatively impact our wellbeing.

To examine the evidence behind the Human Bank Investments, go to "Human Bank Investments Evidence" in the References & Research section at the end of this book.

Human Bank™ 15 Positive Investments

Positive Human Bank™ Investments – Definition.

The 15 Positive Investment actions that deposit life-giving value into the five Human Banks. These investments fill and prosper your Human Bank, and build long-term wellbeing.

Physical Human Bank™

1. Daily, I eat a healthy and nutritious diet (high in fruit & vegetables and low in fat, salt, sugar).

2. Daily, I experience exercise (30-60 mins).

3. Daily, I have self-control to avoid unhealthy coping mechanisms (e.g., excessive eating, excessive drinking, substance use, isolation, excessive screen time, media, or shopping) to deal with stress, anxiety, or negative emotions.

Emotional Human Bank™

1. Each day, I heal emotional upset by processing my feelings, releasing anger, and letting go of bitterness and resentment.

2. Each day, I live in alignment with my authentic 'True' self—my values, beliefs, passions, and purpose.

3. Each day, I express gratitude, recognising that while I may not have everything I want or need, I am content with my life.

Relational Human Bank™

1. Each day, I offer help and support to those in need in my life.

2. Each day, I cultivate deep, authentic relationships with people who uplift and support me.

3. Each day, I have enough money for essentials and spend my money wisely, avoiding debt.

Mental Human Bank™

1. Each day, I practice forgiveness— both for others and for myself.

2. Each day, I live with a sense of meaning and purpose that guides my actions.

3. Each day, I trust in God with things beyond my control.

Soul Human Bank™

1. Each day, I experience a connection to my faith in God that brings me love, peace, and hope.

2. Each day, I live to love and honour God and others with my actions.

3. Each day, I dedicate time to prayer and personal Bible reading.

Human Bank™ 15 Negative Investments

Negative Human Bank™ Investments – Definition.

The 15 Negative Investment actions that drain, deplete, or damage the five Human Banks. These actions withdraw value, diminish long-term wellbeing, and can lead to burnout and the eventual bankruptcy of your Human Bank.

Physical Human Bank™

1. Each day, I do not nourish my body with a balanced diet rich in fruits and vegetables while limiting unhealthy fats, salt, and sugar.

2. Each day, I do not engage in at least 30-60 minutes of physical activity to strengthen my body and improve my wellbeing.

3. Each day, I do not prioritise getting 7-9 hours of restful sleep to restore my energy and health.

Emotional Human Bank™

1. Each day, I struggle to feel safe in the workplace, online, or at home.

2. Each day, I expose myself to dark or harmful media, including violent content, coarse language, negativity, or sexualised material.

3. Each day, I engage in smoking, harming my body and long-term health.

Relational Human Bank™

1. Each day, I engage in addictive behaviours (e.g., excessive social media use, video gaming, online shopping, TV streaming, excessive working, compulsive internet use, pornography, gambling, smoking, drinking, or substance use) that feel out of my control.

2. Each day, I exhibit negative behaviours such as dishonesty, impulsivity, or destructive words and actions that harm myself and others.

3. Each day, I drink alcohol, often in unhealthy amounts (four or more standard drinks).

Mental Human Bank™

1. Each day, I struggle with mental health and with chronic illness challenges such as chronic pain, depression, fear, anxiety, or continual negative thoughts.

2. Each day, I consume excessive amounts (two or more) of caffeine or energy drinks, negatively impacting my health.

3. I regularly misuse prescription or recreational drugs, affecting my wellbeing.

4.

Soul Human Bank™

1. Each day, I choose not to believe in God.

2. Each day, I struggle to find meaning, hope, or purpose, leaving me feeling lost or unfulfilled.

3. Each day, I find it difficult to forgive myself and others, holding onto resentment, hurt, and pain.

In order to help you start your Human Bank journey, I have included a **Human Bank Investment Assessment Template** at the end of this book for your own use. By intentionally investing positively, you will fill up your Human Bank and create a more sustainable, fulfilling and flourishing life. Small, consistent investment actions lead to lasting transformation.

Human Bank™ Investment Impact - Definition

Wellbeing and emotions are intangible and may seem subjective, but examining the return on investment (ROI) through a Human Bank Investment Assessment helps us to measure these things in a tangible, quantifiable way. It is important to consider ROI as this reveals whether our Human Bank experiences **profit** or **loss**.

Human Bank™ Investment Impact - Definition

An evidence-based scoring system that measures the effect of Positive or Negative Investments on the five Human Banks. Each investment yields either a positive or negative return on overall wellbeing and contributes to the health or depletion of your Human Bank.

When we see the positive impact of our investment actions, we can be empowered and inspired to make further positive investments into our Human Bank. Prioritising those investments will help our Human Bank to flourish and prosper. Additionally, when we see the negative investment actions and how they negatively impact our quality of life and overall wellbeing, we will be motivated and inspired to reduce those negative investments that can result in loss and bankruptcy in our Human Bank. So, let's take a look at the impact of positive and negative investments in our Human Bank.

Human Bank™ 15 Positive Investments

Evidence-Based Impact of Positive Investments - Definition

Making intentional positive investments in our physical, emotional, relational, mental, and spiritual wellbeing significantly improves life satisfaction, resilience, and health. Below is an analysis of 15 positive investments and their scientifically supported impacts.

Physical Impact

1. **Healthy & Nutritious Diet**

   - Impact: Reduces the risk of chronic diseases, improves immune function, and supports mental clarity.
   - Evidence: WHO, *Global Nutrition & Health Report*, 2023.

2. **Regular Physical Activity**

   - Impact: Enhances cardiovascular health, boosts energy, and improves mood and stress levels.
   - Evidence: CDC, *Physical Activity and Well-being Study*, 2022.

3. **Self-Control in Coping Mechanisms**

   - Impact: Prevents dependency on harmful coping mechanisms and promotes emotional stability.
   - Evidence: APA, *Self-Control and Emotional Health*, 2023.

Emotional Impact

1. **Processing Emotions & Releasing Negativity**
   - Impact: Increases emotional resilience, reduces anxiety, and improves mental wellbeing.
   - Evidence: NIH, *Emotional Processing and Mental Health*, 2022.
2. **Living in Alignment with True Self**
   - Impact: Brings fulfillment, decreases stress, and enhances overall life satisfaction.
   - Evidence: Harvard Medical School, *Life Alignment Study*, 2023.

3. **Practicing Gratitude**
   - Impact: Improves mood, fosters resilience, and strengthens positive thinking patterns.
   - Evidence: University of California, *Gratitude and Well-being Research*, 2022.

Relational Impact

1. **Helping & Supporting Others**
   - Impact: Builds social connections, increases happiness, and provides a sense of contribution.
   - Evidence: WHO, *Social Connection and Health Report*, 2023.
2. **Building Authentic Relationships**
   - Impact: Enhances emotional support, reduces loneliness, and promotes psychological wellbeing.
   - Evidence: APA, *Mental Health Benefits of Relationships*, 2022.
3. **Financial Responsibility & Debt Management**
   - Impact: Reduces financial and relational stress, increases stability, and promotes responsible money management.
   - Evidence: National Institute of Finance, *Money Management & Well-being*, 2023.

Mental Impact

1. **Practicing Forgiveness**
   - Impact: Lowers stress levels, enhances emotional wellbeing, and improves relationships.
   - Evidence: Mayo Clinic, *The Science of Forgiveness*, 2023.
2. **Living with Meaning & Purpose**
   - Impact: Promotes motivation, personal fulfillment, and a stronger sense of direction.
   - Evidence: APA, *Purpose and Psychological Health Study*, 2023.

3. **Trusting in God**

- Impact: Reduces anxiety, fosters peace of mind, and strengthens faith in overcoming difficulties.

- Evidence: Harvard Divinity School, *Faith and Anxiety Study*, 2023.

Soul (Spiritual) Impact

1. **Experiencing a Connection to Faith in God**

- Impact: Enhances spiritual fulfillment, provides inner peace, and improves emotional stability.

- Evidence: NIH, *Spiritual Health and Mental Resilience*, 2022.

2. **Honouring God & Others Through Actions**

- Impact: Deepens personal relationships, fosters kindness, and strengthens ethical values.

- Evidence: 'Honouring Others and Life Satisfaction', *Theology & Ethics Journal*, 2023.

3. **Dedicating Time to Prayer & Reflection**

- Impact: Supports mental clarity, emotional stability, and spiritual growth.

- Evidence: *Journal of Psychological & Spiritual Practices*, 2023.

Each positive investment strengthens one or more aspects of the Human Bank, contributing to long-term health, happiness, and fulfillment. By prioritising these investments, you can live with meaning, deepen relationships, strengthen faith, and enhance wellbeing.

Human Bank 15 Positive Investments and Impact

Positive Investment	Physical Bank	Emotional Bank	Relational Bank	Mental Bank	Soul Bank	Overall Impact
Physical Bank						
Eating a healthy and nutritious diet daily	5	1	1	1	1	+ 3.8
Engaging in exercise (30-60 min daily)	5	1	1	1	1	+ 3.8
Avoiding unhealthy coping mechanisms	3	3	2	2	1	+ 3.2
Emotional Bank						
Processing emotions & releasing resentment	2	5	2	2	2	+ 3.2
Living in alignment with values & purpose	2	5	2	3	2	+ 3.4
Expressing gratitude daily	1	5	3	2	3	+ 3.4
Relational Bank						
Offering help & support to others	1	2	5	2	2	+ 3.2

Cultivating deep, authentic relationships	1	2	5	2	2	+ 3.2
Managing finances wisely, avoiding debt	2	2	4	2	2	+ 3.0
Mental Bank						
Practicing forgiveness	2	2	2	5	2	+ 3.2
Living with meaning and purpose	1	3	2	5	3	+ 3.4
Trusting in God with things beyond control	1	2	2	3	5	+ 3.2
Soul Bank						
Connecting with faith for peace and hope	1	2	2	3	5	+ 3.2
Loving and honouring God & others with actions	1	2	3	3	5	+ 3.4
Dedicating time to prayer and Bible reading	1	2	2	2	5	+ 3.0

For information on how the Investment Impact Score was calculated, see *The Human Bank™ References & Research* chapter.

Positive Investments Impact Summary

Investing in positive habits across physical, emotional, relational, mental, and spiritual wellbeing significantly enhances overall wellbeing.

Highest Impact Areas:

- Healthy diet (+3.8) and physical activity (+3.8) directly benefits physical health, reduces likelihood of chronic disease and indirectly supports all Human Banks.
- Living with meaning & purpose (+3.4) creates a deep sense of fulfillment and improves mental, emotional, and spiritual wellbeing.
- Living aligned to your values & Beliefs (+3.4) brings a deep peace, sense of value and identity in living your 'true self', and improves overall wellbeing, particularly soul wellbeing.
- Loving God & others (+3.4) brings connection to life and peace to the soul, enabling greater connection and supportive relationships.

Moderate Impact Areas:

- Gratitude (+3.4) enhances joy, emotional stability and relational bonds.
- Practicing forgiveness (+3.2) reduces emotional burden and strengthens mental and relational wellbeing.
- Prayer & personal reflection (+3.0): connection to God cultivates inner peace, emotional healing, and belonging.

- Overall Average Impact: +3.3. Strong positive influence on long-term wellbeing, with mental and spiritual investments having the highest returns.

Human Bank™ 15 Negative Investments and Impact - Definition

Negative investments drain our Human Bank, leading to long-term consequences on physical, emotional, relational, mental, and spiritual wellbeing. Below is an analysis of 15 common negative investments and their documented impacts, backed by evidence.

Physical Impact

1. **Poor Nutrition**

- Impact: Increases the risk of obesity, heart disease, diabetes, and weakens immunity.
- Evidence: WHO, *Global Nutrition Report*, 2023.

2. **Lack of Exercise**

- Impact: Leads to decreased strength, poor circulation, weight gain, and increased stress.
- Evidence: CDC, *Physical Activity Guidelines*, 2022.

3. **Inadequate Sleep**

- Impact: Causes fatigue, poor concentration, reduced immunity, and mental health struggles.
- Evidence: Harvard Medical School, *Sleep Health Study*, 2021.

Emotional Impact

1. **Unsafe Environments**
- Impact: Creates ongoing stress, fear, and anxiety, affecting emotional security.
- Evidence: APA, *Psychological Safety in Environments*, 2023.

2. **Exposure to Harmful Media**

- Impact: Desensitizes the mind, fosters negativity, reduces joy, and increases stress.
- Evidence: WHO, *Media Consumption and Mental Health*, 2022.

3. **Smoking & Substance Use**
- Impact: Damages long-term health, causes addiction, and reduces emotional resilience.
- Evidence: CDC, *Smoking and Chronic Disease Study*, 2021.

Relational Impact

1. **Addictive Behaviours** (e.g., excessive social media, gambling, compulsive shopping)

- Impact: Leads to loss of control, emotional detachment, and neglect of meaningful relationships.

Evidence: NIH, *Internet and Behavioural Addictions,* 2023.

2. **Harmful Words & Actions**
   - Impact: Damages trust, increases conflicts, and isolates individuals from loved ones.

Evidence: 'Impact of Words on Mental Health', *Journal of Social Psychology,* 2022.

3. **Unhealthy Alcohol Consumption**
   - Impact: Affects judgment, affects health, strains relationships, and leads to dependence.

Evidence: *National Institute on Alcohol Abuse and Alcoholism,* 2023.

Mental Impact

1. **Poor Mental Health** (e.g., chronic stress, anxiety, depression)
   - Impact: Increases the risk of depression, anxiety, and emotional distress.

Evidence: WHO, *Global Mental Health Report,* 2023.

2. **Excessive Caffeine or Energy Drinks**
   - Impact: Contributes to restlessness, poor sleep, and long-term health problems.

Evidence: Harvard Health, *Caffeine and Sleep Disruptions,* 2022.

3. **Drug Misuse (prescription or recreational)**
   - Impact: Leads to physical dependence, impaired cognitive function, and poor decision-making.
   - Evidence: National Institute on Drug Abuse, *Drug Impact Study,* 2023.

Soul Impact

1. **Lack of Faith in God**

   - Impact: Can lead to spiritual emptiness, hopelessness, and moral confusion.

   - Evidence: Theology & Faith Review, *Spiritual Fulfillment Study,* 2022.

2. **Absence of Meaning & Purpose**

   - Impact: Increases feelings of depression, lack of motivation, and an inner void.

   Evidence: APA, *Purpose and Mental Health Study,* 2023.

3. **Unforgiveness**

   - Impact: Causes emotional baggage, bitterness, and prolonged suffering.

   Evidence: Mayo Clinic, *Effects of Unforgiveness on Health,* 2022.

Every negative investment has a compounding effect on multiple areas of life. Poor investment choices lead to poor physical health, emotional distress, broken relationships, damage soul health, and a lack of purpose drains the soul. Reversing these negative impacts requires intentional positive investments: nourishing the body, building strong relationships, guarding our soul, and strengthening faith.

Human Bank™ 15 Negative Investments and Impact

Positive Investment	Physical Bank	Emotional Bank	Relational Bank	Mental Bank	Soul Bank	Overall Impact
Physical Bank						
Poor diet (excess sugar, unhealthy fats)	-5	-1	-1	-1	-1	-3.8

Lack of exercise (less than 30 min daily)	-5	-1	-1	-1	-1	-3.8
Poor sleep (less than 7 hours)	-3	-3	-2	-2	-1	-3.2

Emotional Bank

Feeling unsafe in home/work/online	-2	-5	-2	-2	-2	-3.2
Exposure to negative/harmful media	-1	-5	-3	-2	-3	-3.4
Smoking & substance use	-3	-3	-2	-2	-1	-3.0

Relational Bank

Addictive behaviours (social media, gambling)	-1	-2	-5	-2	-2	-3.2
Negative behaviours (lying, impulsivity)	-1	-2	-5	-2	-2	-3.2
Excessive alcohol consumption	-2	-2	-4	-2	-2	-3.0

Mental Bank

Chronic illness & mental health struggles	-2	-2	-2	-5	-2	-3.2
Excessive caffeine or energy drinks	-1	-3	-2	-5	-3	-3.4
Drug misuse (prescription or recreational)	-2	-2	-2	-3	-5	-3.2
Soul Bank						
Choosing not to believe in God	-1	-2	-2	-3	-5	-3.2
Lack of meaning, hope, or purpose	-1	-3	-2	-5	-3	-3.4
Holding onto resentment, unforgiveness	-1	-2	-2	-2	-5	-3.0

For information on how the Investment Impact Score was calculated, see *The Human Bank™ References & Research* chapter.

Negative Investments Impact Summary

Negative habits lead to a decline in overall wellbeing, affecting multiple areas simultaneously.

Highest Negative Impact Areas:

- Unhealthy Diet (-3.8) and lack of exercise (-3.8) directly impacts physical health and can lead to illness and disease, and indirectly impacts overall wellbeing.

- Loss of meaning & purpose (-3.4) creates disconnection from true self and existential distress, increasing mental and emotional suffering.
- Chronic poor mental health (-3.2) affects all dimensions, leading to long-term distress and dysfunction.
- Drug misuse (-3.2) severely impacts physical, mental, emotional, and relational health.

Moderate Negative Impact Areas:

- Unhealthy addictive behaviours (-3.2) leads to emotional instability and dependence on destructive habits.
- Destructive negative behaviours (-3.2) harm relationships, emotional balance, and self-worth.
- Lack of spiritual connection (-3.2) weakens resilience, hope, and overall life satisfaction.
- Overall Impact (-3.3): Consistently negative effects, with mental and relational wellbeing most at risk.

Key Takeaways

1. Relational and Emotional Banks suffer most; negative investments like addictive behaviours, dishonesty, and exposure to harmful media significantly weaken relationships and emotional wellbeing.

2. Mental and Soul Banks are deeply interconnected. Issues like lack of purpose, unforgiveness, and chronic stress show strong connections between spiritual peace and mental resilience.

3. Physical Health is a foundational investment; poor diet, exercise, and sleep reduce energy, impair emotional control, and weaken mental stability, proving that physical investments affect all other areas.

By identifying and addressing these negative investments, you can work towards a healthier, and fulfilling Human Bank. Small changes in daily habits can lead to long-term transformation.

Conclusions

- Positive investments build long-term resilience, meaning, and peace, leading to holistic prosperity in life.

- Negative investments create compounding struggles, particularly in mental and relational wellbeing, often leading to burnout, addiction, and emotional distress.

- Prioritising mental, emotional, and spiritual wellbeing yields the highest impact, reinforcing that true prosperity is about inner fulfillment, not external success.

This matrix provides a clear impact rating for each wellbeing investment, helping prioritise actions with the highest overall benefit and mitigating negative impacts.

Comparing Wellbeing Investment Analysis

What stands out in the comparison of positive and negative investments? Each investment essentially has the same strength impact as its direct opposite. The table below is a powerful visual reminder of the significant impact our investments can make, positively or negatively. It is easy to see how adding one, two, three or more positive or negative investments together will have a major impact on your wellbeing.

Comparative Wellbeing Investment Analysis

Positive and Negative Investment Return

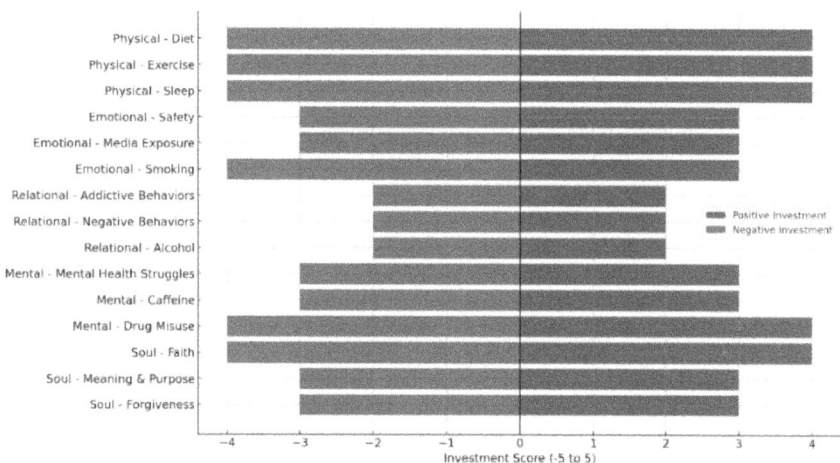

Chapter 6: The Human Bank™ Supply and Demand

Here is a definition of Supply and Demand from Encyclopedia Britannica:

> "Supply and demand, in economics, is the relationship between the quantity of a commodity that producers wish to sell at various prices and the quantity that consumers wish to buy. It is the main model of price determination used in economic theory. The price of a commodity is determined by the interaction of supply and demand in a market." 16

Adam Smith, known as the founder of modern economics, dealt extensively with the topic in his 1776 epic economic work, *The Wealth of Nations*. He noted that there is a correlation between the supply of goods and the price that consumers are prepared to pay for those product and services.

Factors of Production

Obviously, there can be a considerable number of processes and resources required to produce a product or service. Production can be influenced by a number of factors as they affect production capacity, which directly impacts supply availability. Factors of demand include:

- Economic factors

- Social factors

- Environmental factors

When the factors of supply and production are optimal, this leads to increased supply in the market. However, if the factors of supply are down, the supply will not be able to meet the demand of the market. This creates an inequality in supply and demand, potentially leading to market frustrations between producers and consumers. Either the producers cannot sell their goods and services because demand is insufficient or consumers cannot buy because the supply is not available.

Price Equilibrium

When we have both the market producing goods and services, and consumers in the marketplace buying those goods and services, there will be price equilibrium. This is the price at which the quantity of a good or service supplied by producers is equal to the quantity demanded by consumers.

Human Bank™ Supply and Demand Equilibrium – Definition.

The point at which the supply of Human Bank Currency meets the daily demand placed on a person's life indicating a state of balance. At equilibrium, the deposits (investments) into the five Human Banks the withdrawals (demands), resulting in stability, sustainability, and wellbeing.

Human Bank™ Supply and Demand – Definition.

A concept for evaluating the supply of and the demand for our Human Bank Currencies highlighting whether there is oversupply, undersupply, or equilibrium. It reveals the balance (or imbalance) between what is available in our wellbeing reserves and what is being withdrawn daily across the five P.E.R.M.S. Human Banks.

We can take this concept of supply and demand and apply it to our Human Bank concept. It specifically relates to the five currencies: Energy, Joy, Love, Peace and Freedom. Let's create a scenario in which we apply the above concept to the Human Banks. In this scenario, all five of the Human Banks have a maximum currency of 10 units.

Human Bank™ Currency:

- Physical Human Bank™ currency is **Energy**   10

- Emotional Human Bank™ currency is **Joy**   10

- Relational Human Bank™ currency is **Love**   10

- Mental Human Bank™ currency is **Peace**   10

- Soul Human Bank™ currency is **Freedom**   10

Human Bank Demand and Supply - daily scenario

Human Bank Currency HBC	HB Currency Available Balance	Demand High Work Hours	Demand High Caffeine Intake	Demand Work/ Personal Relationship	Supply Daily Exercise -30 mins	Demand Poor Daily Diet	HB C Supply/ Demand Balance
Physical - Energy	10	-4	-3	-3	+3	-4	-7
Emotional - Joy	10	-3	-2	-3	+2	-3	-9
Relational - Love	10	-2	-1	-4	+2	-2	-7
Mental - Peace	10	-4	-3	-3	+3	-3	-10
Soul - Freedom	10	-3	-1	-4	+3	-2	-7

Demand Impacts

Here are some of the evidence-based impacts on these life factors:

- Physical stress
- Emotional stress
- Relationships stress

- Jitters & anxiety
- Irritability
- Restlessness

- Mental stress
- Soul stress
- Work stress
- Overwhelm

- Mood impact
- Low energy for connection
- Cognitive fog
- Less time for relationships

Imagine experiencing the impacts of demand every day, only they keep compounding, bringing you to the point of feeling exasperated, not being able to think clearly, lacking energy and not being able to function properly. Sadly, that is what happens to millions of people around the world and thousands will likely experience it today!

Why? because their Human Bank is empty, bankrupt and trading with an increasing liability: demand is greater than supply. Do you have the Human Bank Currency (HBC) to meet the daily demands of your life?

The optimal goal for our Human Bank Currencies are:

- **Physical currency** – Supplying our daily demand for **energy.**

- **Emotional currency** – Supplying our daily demand for **joy.**

- **Relational currency** – Supplying our daily demand for **love.**

- **Mental currency** – Supplying our daily demand for **peace.**

- **Soul currency** – Supplying our daily demand for **freedom.**

The tables on the next page provide three scenarios showing the daily demand of our Human Bank Currency:

Human Bank™ Currency - Demand and Supply

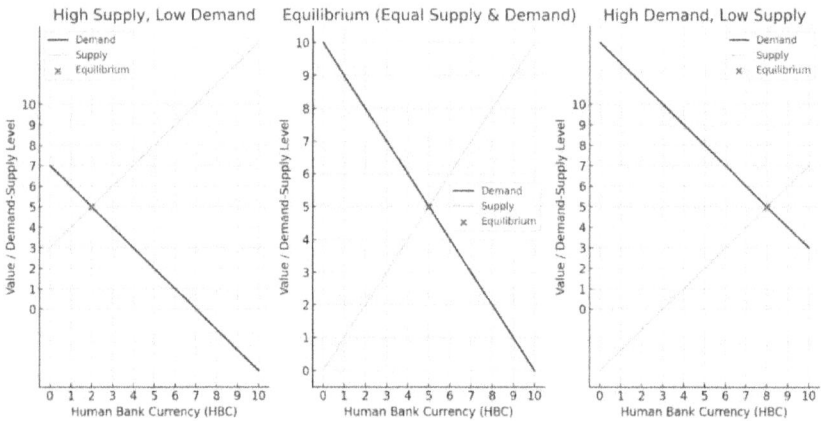

Chart 1. HBC High Supply, Low Demand → Excess supply of HBC more than adequate to meet our daily demands = inefficiency.

Chart 2. HBC Equilibrium (Equal Supply & Demand) → The supply of our HBC meets our daily demands = equilibrium.

Chart 3. HBC High Demand, Low Supply → Loss and scarcity of our HBC, insufficient to meet daily demands = high stress.

The above tables powerfully visualise the concept of demand and supply in the Human Bank and how the five currencies are needed to meet the demands of daily life.

Breakdown of Chart 1

This scenario illustrates that when Human Bank Currency is greater than the daily output demands, it results in the Human Bank being in profit, with excess currency to invest. In this case, our Human Banks are operationally, viable and sustainable. However, this can sometimes result in an inefficient use of resources.

Breakdown of Chart 2

In this scenario, there is an equilibrium between supply and demand. Supply of Human Bank Currency equals the demand of Human Bank Currency, thus the banks operate sustainably and meet output requirements. It shows maximum efficiency, with all currency being expended and fully utilised. This minimises stress, as there is neither an excess of demand neither is there profit – excess Human Bank Currency.

Breakdown of Chart 3

The Human Bank Currency supply is inadequate to meet the daily demands of the human Banks, thus resulting in one or more of the Human Banks being in deficit, unable to supply demand-. This is not viable in its operation and not sustainable.

This inadequacy and inequality causes stress on whichever Human Bank is experiencing the deficit. If this continues it can result in bankruptcy of the Human bank; that is, being unable to meet the demands of life. There are three possibilities in this scenario:

1. We seek to use Counterfeit Currency; quick fixes to get us through the day. Generally, we turn to stimulants and substances: caffeine, alcohol, or drugs to meet our demand, seeking to getting through anyway we can. This results in **disparity/loss**;

2. We reduce the demands and thus move closer to the demands meeting our supply: **equilibrium**. Or;

3. We seek to invest to increase the supply of Human Bank Currency to meet demand, resulting in a **surplus/profit**.

Human Bank™ Currency: Supply & Demand Index HBCSDI Impact Matrix - Definition

An evidence-based scoring and diagnostic matrix that measures the supply and demand of Human Bank Currency across the five Human Banks. It identifies areas of balance, oversupply, or deficit, providing insight into a person's overall wellbeing and highlighting which Human Banks need intentional investment.

It helps individuals:

- Identify surplus (oversupply),

- Recognise deficit (undersupply),

- Confirm equilibrium (balanced supply and demand),

...in each Human Bank offering insight into which domains are under strain from high demand and low supply, and highlighting where intentional reinvestment is most needed to restore wellbeing.

Demand & Supply Life Factors

Let's look at an example of what demands and supplies an average person might have in a typical day. In this scenario we have the following wellbeing life factors:

1. Daily 10 hours of work per day.

2. Excessive caffeine intake 2+ drinks per day

3. Moderate to high work/personal relationships demands

4. Daily exercise of 30 mins

5. Poor diet low in nutrition high in fats, salt, sugar.

We will run this scenario over five days to see the compound impact when the same wellbeing life factors are applied. Please note: in this scenario the five Human Banks start with the maximum Currency or 10 units.

To help us qualify the demand and supply of our life factors on our Human Bank let's develop our Supply and Demand Impact Matrix. The following Supply and Demand Impact ratings are evidence based. For the methodology and scoring of the *Human Bank™ Currency: Supply & Demand Index (HBCSDI)*, refer to the *Human Bank™ References & Research* section.

Day 1: Human Bank™ Currency: Supply & Demand Index HBCSDI Matrix 1

Human Bank Currency HBC	HB Currency Available Balance	Demand High Work Hours	Demand High Caffeine Intake	Demand Work/ Personal Relationship	Supply Daily Exercise -30 mins	Demand Poor Daily Diet	HBC Supply/ Demand Balance
Physical - **Energy**	10	-3	-2	-2	4	-3	4
Emotional – **Joy**	10	-2	-3	-3	3	-2	3
Relational – **Love**	10	-2	-1	-4	2	-1	4
Mental - **Peace**	10	-4	-3	-3	3	-2	1
Soul - **Freedom**	10	-2	-1	-2	4	-3	6

Summary:

This scenario covers five common lifestyle factors in the life of the average employee.

- To begin with, all five Human Bank Currencies had adequate supply for the daily demands (profit).
- There was a **supply** of HBC through 30 minutes of exercise. This highlights that we can positively invest back into Human Bank through positive investments.
- Interestingly; the supply of HBC through 30 minutes of exercise kept the HBC balance in profit!

Now let's look at the next day, carrying over the Human Bank Currency Supply/Demand Balance from the previous day. **In Matrix 1 we had full currency (10) to begin with in all Human Bank Currencies.** and now the previous day's end balance becomes the second day's opening currency balance.

Day 2: Human Bank™ Currency: Supply & Demand Index (HBCSDI) Matrix 2

Human Bank Currency HBC	HB Currency Available Balance	Demand High Work Hours	Demand High Caffeine Intake	Demand Work/ Personal Relationship	Supply Daily Exercise -30 mins	Demand Poor Daily Diet	HBC Supply/ Demand Balance
Physical - **Energy**	4	-3	-2	-2	4	-3	0
Emotional - **Joy**	3	-2	-3	-3	3	-2	-4
Relational - **Love**	4	-2	-1	-4	2	-1	-2
Mental - **Peace**	1	-4	-3	-3	3	-2	-8
Soul - **Freedom**	6	-2	-1	-2	4	-3	2

What stands out to you? Do you see a pattern? Perhaps you noticed that currency levels **do not** reset back to 10 every day and start over again as if it's Groundhog Day. This highlights the compounding effect supply and demand has on the following day. In other words, demands on the supply of Human Bank Currency not only outweighed the investments/deposits but is now pushing our Human Bank Currency into negative balance. Now, three of our Human Bank Currencies are in deficit with only one on zero.

This means that the person would be experiencing the significant impacts of having low levels of (or no) energy, joy, love, peace and freedom. How would that be impacting their life?

Let's continue to Day 3, keeping the same life factors and using the previous day's HBC balance.

Day 3: Human Bank™ Currency: Supply & Demand Index (HBCSDI) Matrix 3

Human Bank Currency HBC	HB Currency Available Balance	Demand High Work Hours	Demand High Caffeine Intake	Demand Work/ Personal Relationship	Supply Daily Exercise -30 mins	Demand Poor Daily Diet	HBC Supply/ Demand Balance
Physical - Energy	0	-3	-2	-2	4	-3	-6
Emotional - Joy	-4	-2	-3	-3	3	-2	-11
Relational - Love	-2	-2	-1	-4	2	-1	-8
Mental - Peace	-8	-4	-3	-3	3	-2	-17
Soul - Freedom	-2	-2	-1	-2	4	-3	-2

What are your observations of the Supply/Demand balance? What do you think some of the impacts the Supply/Demand balance would have on a person's life? They would start to see significant impacts on their wellbeing, flowing through, and compounding each other.

Consider long work hours as an example: high caffeine intake to sustain energy and concentration, leads to poor sleep due to being highly stimulated by caffeine, which in turn results in the person not sleeping well, waking up tired and irritated, and therefore feeling like they need more caffeine (Foreign Currency) to get by. This increases poor sleep by being over stimulated and the cycle continues.

Day 4: Human Bank™ Currency: Supply & Demand Index (HBCSDI) Matrix 4

Human Bank Currency HBC	HBC Balance	Demand High Work Hours	Demand High Caffeine Intake	Demand Work/ Personal Relations	Supply Exercise -30 mins	Demand Poor Diet Intake	Demand Poor Sleep Quality	HBC Supply/ Demand Balance
Physical - Energy	-6	-3	-2	-2	4	-3	-3	-15
Emotional - Joy	-11	-2	-3	-3	3	-2	-3	-21
Relational - Love	-8	-2	-1	-4	2	-1	-2	-16
Mental - Peace	-17	-4	-3	-3	3	-2	-4	-30
Soul - Freedom	-2	-2	-1	-2	4	-3	-2	-8

Day 4 includes another life factor: poor sleep. This has largely been contributed to by excess caffeine intake which in turn stimulates the body's function and overrides the sleep cycle. Secondly, work stress resulted in adrenaline in the system. This also had a significant impact on Human Bank Currency and further pushed the Human Bank Currencies into deficit.

Day 5: Human Bank™ Currency: Supply & Demand Index HBCSDI Matrix 5

Human Bank Currency HBC	HBC Balance	Demand High Work Hours	Demand High Caffeine Intake	Demand High Relation- ship	Supply Daily Exercise - 30 mins	Demand Poor Daily Diet	Demand Poor Daily Sleep	Demand Poor Coping Methods	HBC Supply/ Demand Balance
Physical - Energy	-15	-3	-2	-2	4	-3	-3	-3	-27

Emotional - Joy	-21	-2	-3	-3	3	-2	-3	-5	**-36**
Relational - Love	-16	-2	-1	-4	2	-1	-2	-2	**-26**
Mental - Peace	-30	-4	-3	-3	3	-2	-4	-5	**-46**
Soul - Freedom	-8	-2	-1	-2	4	-3	-2	-4	**-18**
Total Impact	-90								**-153**

Day 5 introduces negative coping mechanisms/methods. The individual is not coping at all. Lack of sleep for days, no energy resulting in work stress, relational stress and mental stress. This flows out of not coping with having sufficient Human Bank Currency to meet daily life demands. With their currency overdrawn and their Human Banks in deficit, the individual resorts to another external negative coping mechanism (**Counterfeit Currency**) such as drinking more alcohol. This means they are now totalling two Counterfeit Currencies (alcohol and caffeine) which further negatively compound the disparity of Supply and Demand of their Human Bank. Ultimately, this results in an increased sense of hopelessness, depression, overwhelm and anxiety. **This course of action is not sustainable, and if these life factors continue a significant life crisis is imminent.**

Below is the Updated Human Bank Currency: Supply Demand Curve for this individual, showing the disparity between Supply and Demand.

This is a helpful visual of the Supply and Demand concept and how it applies to a Human Bank. We see some significant impact flow through to the currency levels of the Human Bank, reaching double digit negative figures. As you can see, the results are shocking, and devastating in their impact. This is a serious health, wellbeing and life crisis. Surely, this is not how life is meant to be lived!

Human Bank Currency Demand and Supply Curve

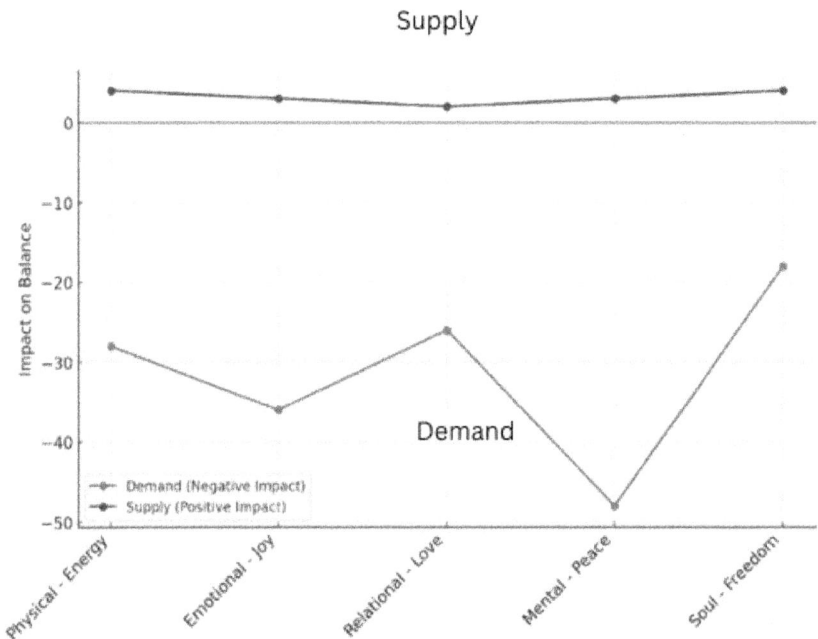

Supply

This is a helpful visual of the Supply and Demand concept and how it applies to a Human Bank. We see some significant impact flow through to the currency levels of the Human Bank, reaching double digit negative figures. As you can see, the results are shocking, and devastating in their impact. This is a serious health, wellbeing and life crisis. Surely, this is not how life is meant to be lived!

The consequences that the person would be experiencing would have a significant impact on their lifestyle function, cognitive ability, daily productivity, and relationships, resulting in severe stress, exhaustion and anxiety.

The Compound Effect

Let's examine the effects the life factors had on the individual:

- **High Daily Work Hours (demand):** This resulted in feeling run down, with low energy levels daily. Not being able to cope with the demands increases stress.
- **Demand - Excessive Caffeine Intake (demand):** Low energy levels resulted in the individual turning to caffeine to supplement low energy

levels. As it is a short-term fix and Counterfeit Currency, this is reported as a demand.

- **Daily Work/Personal Relationship (demand):** As the person was experiencing low energy levels (feeling tired and tense) this translated into stressed interactions and communication in both work and personal relationships. The resulting relational stress added to the existing work stress, compounding into multiple stressors.
- **Exercising for 30 minutes (supply):** This helped reduce some stress and invest some health and wellbeing back into the Human Bank.
- **Poor Diet (demand):** Long work hours left the individual tired and time poor, reducing the time and effort they were willing to spend on preparing healthy meals. The resulting poor diet had a significant negative impact on the individual, as the body did not receive the nourishment required to energise the body for the daily outputs. This further exasperated low energy levels, decreasing productivity, increasing stress and the need for Counterfeit Currency: Caffeine. Result: not having capacity to cope with mounting multiple stressors, significantly affecting physical, emotional, relational, mental and soul wellbeing.
- **Poor Sleep (demand):** One of the most significant life factors is sleep. It is a time when the body rests and heals, preparing for the day ahead. If this process is compromised so, is our wellbeing. The high caffeine intake significantly impeded the quality and also quantity of the individual's sleep. Stress and anxiety relating to their work situation contributed to the individual having difficulty going to sleep at night. When the body lacks adequate sleep, it does not have that chance to replenish and we start the next day lacking sufficient energy. As we can see in the demand supply matrix, this keeps compounding daily, impacting all Human Banks and currencies.
- **Poor Coping Methods (demand):** The progressive deterioration of wellbeing and experiencing deficit in all Human Banks resulted in the individual turning to negative coping mechanisms to try to "get by".
    - Nights were the time for switching off, providing an escape with hours of binge-watching tv and drinking alcohol.

When we do not take the time or know how to invest into our Human Bank, we will often turn to Counterfeit Currency or negative coping methods. Sadly, this does not give us what we truly need to prosper in our physical, emotional, relational, mental and soul wellbeing, and our longing for energy, joy, love, peace and freedom continues.

Michael J. Smith

This individual was negative in all Human Bank Currencies. This means that:

- Physical Bank Currency is Energy; **they were not experiencing physical energy.**
- Emotional Bank Currency is Joy; **they were not experiencing joy in their emotions.**
- Relational Bank Currency is Love; **they were not experiencing love in their relationships.**
- Mental Bank Currency is Peace; **they were not experiencing peace of mind.**
- Soul Bank Currency is Freedom; **they were not experiencing freedom in their soul.**

Currency	The Compound Effect Impact
Energy	Tired, lacking energy for daily work and personal life.
Joy	Being exhausted, stress took away all joy, and daily life was a tiring obligation.
Love	Exhaustion and other stresses added to relational stress, conflict and feeling unloved.
Peace	Anxiety or pressure replaced peace and influenced actions and behaviour professionally and personally.
Freedom	The individual was exhausted in a daily cycle of draining work and poor sleep; they felt trapped and lacked the freedom to break out of this cycle.

Imagine if this played out day after day, week after week. Consider:

- What impact would it have on the person?

- How would it affect their **physical, emotional, relational, mental and soul wellbeing**?

- How would they try to cope and manage?

- How would their relationships be affected professionally and personally?

Human Bank Currency Deficits

When we lack Human Bank Currency to meet our daily demands, it creates deficits across our five Human Banks, leading to depletion of our overall wellbeing. Such Demand Deficit impacts could include:

1. Physical Bank Currency Energy Deficit

- Depletion of Energy: we feel drained and unable to function optimally.
- Impact: Physical exhaustion, chronic stress, or even illness.

2. Emotional Bank Currency Joy Deficit

- Depletion of Joy: We lose excitement, hope and meaning.
- Impact: Emotional exhaustion, Anxiety, mood swings, emotional numbness, or burnout.

3. Relational Bank Currency Love Deficit

- Depletion of Love: We lose connection and support from other people weakens, leading to loneliness.
- Impact: Relational exhaustion, isolation, strained relationships, lack of trust, or conflicts.

4. Mental Bank Currency Peace Deficit

- Depletion of Peace: Inner clarity and calmness are replaced by stress and chaos.
- Impact: Mental exhaustion, brain fog, poor decision-making, lack of focus, confusion or mental exhaustion.

5. Soul Bank Currency Freedom Deficit

- Depletion of Freedom: We feel trapped in circumstances, lacking the capacity to change, lacking fulfillment and direction.
- Impact: Soul exhaustion, loss of purpose, spiritual emptiness, disconnection from true self and God.

When all these banks run low, it creates a pattern of depletion that has a compound effect on every aspect of life. Replenishing our Human Bank Currency is essential to maintaining balance, wellbeing, and flourishing in our Human Banks. The state of Human Banks in a constant state of loss, deficit and bankruptcy could be described in economic terms as "Bank Failure".

Human Bank Currency: Supply & Demand Index (HBCSDI) Impact Matrix description.

HBC	Energy	Joy	Love	Peace	Freedom
High supply/ low demand	Excess Energy	Excess Joy	Excess Love	Excess Peace	Excess Freedom
Equal Supply = Demand	Adequate Energy	Adequate Joy	Adequate Love	Adequate Peace	Adequate Freedom
Low supply /high demand	Low Energy	Low Joy	Low Love	Low Peace	Low Freedom
	Lethargic Un - productive Stressed Burnout Frustrated	Depressed, Sad Hope-less Oppression	Unloved Unloving Relational- tension	Anxiety, Fear, Insecurity Worry Upset	Trapped, Restricted Depressed Captive Slave

(HBCSDI) Impact Matrix description

In this Impact Matrix, we can see the impacts of High Supply, Equal Supply and Low Supply of our Human Bank Currency. Think of it as further incentive to invest in our Human Bank so that we have adequate Human Bank Currency:

- Providing adequate energy for our daily life.

- Providing adequate joy for our daily life.

- Providing adequate love for our daily life.

- Providing adequate peace for our daily life.

- Providing adequate freedom for our daily life.

How would life feel? How would life be different? Imagine if you had an oversupply of Human Bank Currency:

- Excess Energy, Joy, Love, Peace and Freedom in your daily life.

Imagine how this would empower you, day after day and week after week. Consider the overall impact it would have on your life. Specifically:

- How would your professional and personal relationships be affected?

There is hope for change, hopefully that encourages you to starts by reducing the demands on your wellbeing and increasing investments and currency supply to your Human Bank so that you can prosper in your Human Bank and prosper in life.

Chapter 7: Human Bank™ Bankruptcy (Bank Failure)

We begin this chapter with a definition of *Bank Failure*:

> "A **bank failure** occurs when a bank is unable to meet its obligations to its depositors or other creditors because it has become insolvent too illiquid to meet its liabilities." 17

Similarly, we can experience **Human Bank failure**; depletion, exhaustion, and eventual breakdown, with our Human Banks being unable to meet their daily withdrawals and obligations. Just as we experience financial stress when we don't have enough money to meet the demands of daily living, we experience physical, emotional, relational, mental or spiritual stress when we don't have the Human Bank Currency in one or multiple of our P.E.R.M.S. Human Banks.

Human Bank™ Insolvency Bankruptcy - Definition

A critical state of depletion in which one or more of the five Human Banks Physical, Emotional, Relational, Mental, or Soul becomes chronically drained due to repeated negative investments and insufficient replenishment. This condition often results in burnout, emotional distress, spiritual disconnection, or overall wellbeing collapse.

Collective Stress

When these stresses are combined, it can place significant burden on our Human Bank's currency function and whole-life wellbeing. There is an economic term, **market failure**, which results when supply cannot meet the demand. Here is a definition:

> "**Market failure** refers to the inefficient allocation of resources that occurs when individuals acting in rational self-interest produce a sub-optimal outcome." 18

Let's for a moment consider inefficient allocation of resources. It means that we have the resources (Human Bank Currency) but we spent or perhaps invested it unwisely rather than optimally.

People often experience this as burnout, stress, overwhelm, anxiety, or depression. These are symptoms of Human Bank market failure. Chronic illness is often the result of being deficit in our Human Bank and wellbeing.

Imagine a person faces constant work demands but lacks the energy to meet them. In effect, their Human Bank is bankrupt if they cannot supply physical currency (energy). The disparity between supply and demand creates a market failure in our Human Bank.

We need to understand that there are demands on our Human Bank Currency (energy, joy, love, peace, freedom) every day and if we do not have the supply to meet that demand, the resulting deficit causes physical, emotional, relational, mental, and spiritual stress, reduced quality of life, and increased likelihood of chronic disease. All as a result of bankruptcy of our Human Bank.

To prevent this, we must:

1. Monitor withdrawals: reduce unnecessary expenditures of our Human Bank Currency (HBC), and;

2. Increase deposits: make intentional investments into our Human Bank Currency (HBC).

By maintaining a healthy Human Bank, we can avoid deficit, increase surplus, and ultimately thrive and flourish in our daily life. This brings increased peace, joy, happiness and feeling like we are coping in our day. That is my heart's desire for you. I pray that this has been a blessing to you, and that it will become a lifelong principle for you to flourish in your Human Bank.

Chapter 8: The Human Bank™ Profit & Loss

How does our Human Bank result in profit or loss? It is by the investments we make. In Chapter 5 we learned about the 15 Positive and 15 Negative Human Bank Investments. The below Profit and Loss Statement adds the value of each investment so that you can calculate your Profit or Loss.

Why is this important?

The whole concept of the Human Bank is that we quantify our wellbeing. Wellbeing is very subjective, and putting it into a quantifiable framework helps us identify the negative investments deducting from our Human Bank and the Positive Investments that add wellbeing. This allows us to see if we are in Profit or Loss in our wellbeing. With this tool, you can start investing to prosper in your Human Bank.

Human Bank™ Profit & Loss Statement - Definition

An outcome determined by the Human Bank™ Investment Assessment, which evaluates whether your life is currently in profit or loss across the five Human Banks - Physical, Emotional, Relational, Mental, and Soul. It measures the net effect of your positive and negative investments to reveal whether you are replenishing (in profit) or depleting (in loss) your overall wellbeing.

To assess you Human Bank Profit and Loss complete the *"Human Bank™ Investment Assessment" (Human Bank™ 15 Positive Investments & Human Bank™ 15 Negative Investments)* in the *Human Bank™ Resources* section at the back of the book.

Net Human Bank Balance = Profits – Losses

Profit — Identify the banks that are generating profit and maintain your investments in those banks.

Balanced - This means if a person invests equally in positive and negative factors, they break even—neither in profit or loss.

Loss - Resulting from negative investments being greater the Positive investments.

To truly prosper, positive investments must outweigh negative investments.

Human Bank™ Profit & Loss Statement - example

Category	Profitable Investments (Income)	Loss Investments (Expenses)	Net Profit/Loss
Physical Bank	12	-14	-2
Emotional Bank	13	-12	1
Relational Bank	10	-11	-1
Mental Bank	13	-13	0
Soul Bank	10	-9	1
Total Income & Expenses	**58**	**-59**	**-1 (Slight Deficit)**

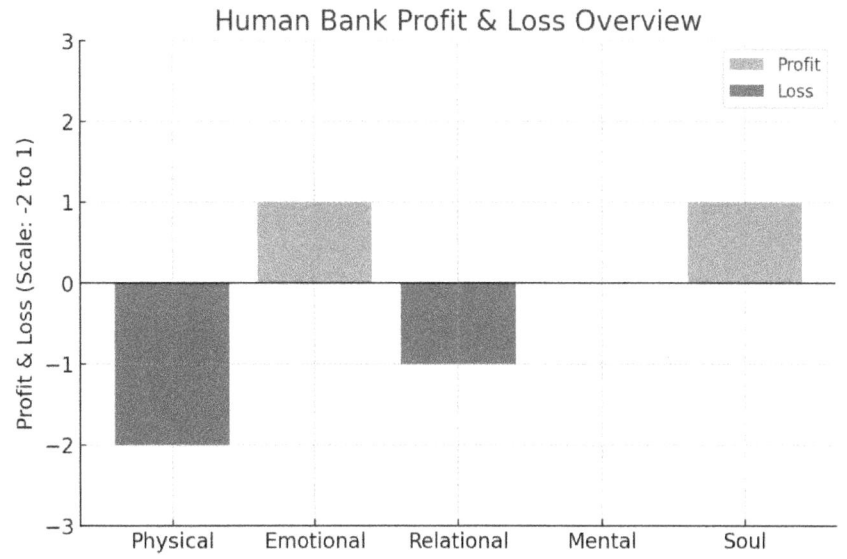

Human Bank Profit & Loss Overview

Key Takeaways

- The overall balance is -1, meaning this person is in a Human Bank deficit.

- Top Negative Impact Areas:

    o Relational Wellbeing (-1 Net Balance) → Moderate impact on relationships, limited experience of being loved or being loving.

    o Physical Health (-2 Net Balance) → Poor diet, lack of exercise, and insufficient sleep affecting wellbeing.

Let me share an experience I had while writing *Human Bank*. I was sitting in a café with my laptop and stopped to reflect on a conversation I overheard in which a hard-working man was describing his life, work, and family struggles. "Working 70 hrs per week, I have nothing left, I feel like leaning back on the couch and doing nothing, but I can't because my kids need me, my kids are a mess that I need to clean up."

My heart went out to the man. I felt his pain and the heaviness of his heart. He was just now looking for a solution, now that he was at breaking point. It was only then that the mess, complexity and pain were significant enough to move him to relieve the situation. When the pain is too great, the cost is too significant. The longer the problem goes for and the more complex it becomes, the more it takes to bring, life, resolution, and profit into that circumstance and area of life.

I do not think it was a coincidence that the man shared his desperate situation as I was writing about the desperate need of people and the desperate need to help them.

We urgently need to take a snapshot of our lives. Where are we at right now? We are not designed to endure physical, emotional, relational, mental or spiritual burnout and breakdown.

If we are to avoid such circumstances we need to analyse and understand our current Human Bank and our need to invest positively now!

Chapter 9: The Human Bank™ Balance Sheet

The balance sheet is the measure of the assets and liabilities of an organisation.

- Assets are what you **own**
- Liabilities are what you **owe**

If the liabilities are greater than the assets the business is potentially insolvent, unable to meet its current liabilities and service its debt. Conversely, when the business has assets greater than its liabilities, the organisation is sustainable and viable to continue operating.

If a business doesn't have a ready supply of cash/capital it is in crisis if it cannot meet day-to-day expenses. This is called a cash flow shortage. Cash flow is the life blood of a business. Cash flow to a business is like carbon dioxide to a plant; it can survive for a time without sun and water, but take away CO_2 and it cannot breathe and will die very quickly.

Assets are important because they indicate stability; the business can convert assets to currency.

Human Bank™ Balance Sheet - Definition

A snapshot of an individual's overall wellbeing, showing the current state of their Human Bank by comparing assets (available Human Bank Currency) to liabilities (debt or deficits in Human Bank Currency). It reflects the balance or imbalance of each of the five Human Banks.

Assets (Profitable Investments)

Human Bank™ Asset - Definition

A positive investment, behaviour, or decision that creates Human Bank Currency (profit) within a person's Human Bank. Assets replenish and build up the Human Bank adding Energy, Joy, Love, Peace, or Freedom currency across the five Human Banks. They enhance overall wellbeing and expand a person's capacity to invest positively.

Human Bank™ Liability - Definition

A negative pattern, behaviour, or decision that creates a debt or burden within a person's Human Bank. Liabilities deplete Human Bank Currency across the five Human Banks and reduce a person's overall wellbeing and capacity to invest positively.

To assess you Human Bank Balance Sheet complete the *"Human Bank™ Investment Assessment" (Human Bank™ 15 Positive Investments & Human Bank™ 15 Negative Investments)* in the *Human Bank™ Resources* section at the back of the book.

Key Insights:

- If Assets > Liabilities, the individual experiences healthy, positive wellbeing growth.

- If Liabilities > Assets, the individual is in a wellbeing deficit.

- The goal is to increase Profitable Investments, producing Assets while reducing Loss liabilities Investments for a strong and prosperous Human Bank.

Human Bank™ Balance Sheet (Based on Profit & Loss Statement) Example.

This **Balance Sheet** reflects the net impact of **Profitable Investments (Assets)** and **Loss Investments (Liabilities)** on overall wellbeing.

Category	Assets (Profitable Investments)	Liabilities (Loss Investments)	Net Worth (Balance)
Physical Bank	12	-14	-2
Emotional Bank	13	-12	1
Relational Bank	10	-11	-1

Mental Bank	13	-13	0
Soul Bank	10	-9	1
Total Assets & Liabilities	58	-59	**-1 (Slight deficit)**

Key Insights from this example:

- Balanced Human Bank: the net balance is only -1, meaning the individual is close to breaking even.
- Emotional & Soul Investments: Faith, gratitude, and emotional healing help stabilise the balance. Biggest Loss Area: Physical Health (-2 net balance) → Poor sleep, lack of exercise, and unhealthy diet have the highest negative impact.

How is your Balance Sheet? Is your Human Bank Insolvent? Do your liabilities exceed your assets?

For the Human Bank to fail (become insolvent) our liabilities must be greater than our Human Bank Assets. Meaning, we do not have the currency to repay our Human Bank Liabilities. This can result in bankruptcy; bank failure.

Are you balanced between neutral liabilities and assets? In other words, do you have equal amounts of assets and liabilities?

Or, do you have a positive, healthy balance sheet where you have assets greater than liabilities? In other words, you have surplus Human Bank Currency for what you need daily, so that you are in surplus (profit)? If so, your Human Bank is stable, strong, and healthy. This enables you to grow and develop physically, emotionally, relationally, mentally, and spiritually. In short, you have options! Investment options that are beneficial and build positively in your life and others.

Consider this a call to be a **wise investor**, to invest in daily activities that invest positively into your Human Bank, so we make a profitable return.

Chapter 10: The Human Bank™ Return on Investment

Let's progress to the return on our investments. Every action in life has a cause and effect. Something never equals nothing. Every action has meaning and a consequence which will either be positive or negative. It is rare that a positive action can produce a negative effect, and similarly unusual that a negative action can produce a positive outcome.

Human Bank™ Return on Investment (ROI) - Definition

The resulting profit or loss determined through the Human Bank™ Investment Assessment. It applies evidence-based wellbeing impact to each investment across the five Human Banks revealing how daily choices either contribute to or diminish overall wellbeing.

Rather than forfeiting future wellbeing, you can make restorative choices receive a **compounding return** in overall health, satisfaction, and spiritual vitality. This model affirms that every positive action today is an investment that multiplies life and wellbeing tomorrow.

With that in mind, let's take a look at our investments and their return:

Human Bank™ Return on Positive Investment Model - Definition

The Human Bank™ Return on Positive Investment Model reveals the evidence-based value gained from intentional, life-giving wellbeing choices. Each Positive Investment deposits Human Bank Currency such as Energy, Joy, Love, Peace, or Freedom into one of the five Human Banks

Bank	Positive Investment	Impact on Wellbeing
Physical Bank		

Bank	Positive Investment	Impact on Wellbeing
	Healthy & Nutritious Diet	Reduces chronic disease risk, boosts immunity, supports mental clarity
	Regular Physical Activity	Enhances heart health, energy, mood, and reduces stress
	Self-Control in Coping	Prevents unhealthy behaviours, stabilises emotional health
Emotional Bank		
	Processing Emotions & Letting Go	Improves resilience, reduces anxiety, enhances mental wellbeing
	Living in Alignment with True Self	Increases fulfillment and reduces stress
	Practicing Gratitude	Improves mood, builds resilience, supports positive thinking
Relational Bank		
	Helping & Supporting Others	Boosts happiness, social connection, and sense of purpose
	Building Authentic Relationships	Improves emotional support, reduces loneliness
	Financial Responsibility & Debt Avoidance	Reduces relational stress, promotes financial and emotional stability
Mental Bank		

Bank	Positive Investment	Impact on Wellbeing
	Practicing Forgiveness	Reduces stress, improves emotional health and relationships
	Living with Meaning & Purpose	Promotes fulfilment and strong life direction
	Trusting in God	Reduces anxiety, builds peace and inner strength
Soul Bank		
	Experiencing Connection to Faith	Enhances peace, spiritual fulfilment, emotional balance
	Honouring God & Others	Deepens relationships, fosters kindness, strengthens values
	Dedicating Time to Prayer & Bible Reading	Supports clarity, emotional stability, and spiritual growth

I want to focus specifically on the 15 Negative Investments from Chapter 5 as they produce impacts that people generally are not aware of (which is why they make those negative investments).

Human Bank™ Return on Negative Investment Model - Definition

The Human Bank™ Return on Negative Investment Model reveals the evidence-based loss incurred from repeated unhealthy or self-damaging wellbeing behaviours. Each Negative Investment withdraws valuable Human Bank Currency—such as Energy, Joy, Love, Peace, or Freedom—from one or more of the five Human Banks.

Positive Investment Impact on Wellbeing

Physical Bank

Poor diet (high fat, sugar, salt, low nutrients)	Increases risk of obesity, cardiovascular diseases, and mental health issues
Lack of daily physical activity	Contributes to obesity, musculoskeletal disorders, and psychological issues
Poor sleep (less than 7-9 hours)	Leads to weakened immune system, obesity, and substance abuse

Emotional Bank

Feeling unsafe at work, online, or home	Associated with chronic stress, leading to mental health problems and medical issues
Exposure to harmful media content	Linked to mental health problems, including depression and anxiety
Smoking or self-harm behaviours	Increases the risk of chronic diseases and mental health issues

Relational Bank

Addictive behaviours (excessive media, shopping, gambling, etc.)	Associated with mental health problems and substance abuse
Negative behaviours (dishonesty, impulsivity, destructive actions)	Can lead to social and psychological problems
Alcohol consumption (unhealthy levels)	Leads to various health issues, including liver disease and heart problems

Mental Bank

Poor Mental Health	Increases the risk of depression, anxiety, and emotional distress.

Excessive caffeine/energy drinks	Linked to mental health problems and substance abuse
Misusing prescription or recreational drugs	Increases the risk of addiction and mental health issues

Soul Bank

Choosing not to believe in God	May affect psychological well-being and sense of purpose
Struggling with meaning, hope, and purpose	Associated with mental health problems and premature death
Holding onto resentment, struggling with forgiveness	Linked to mental health problems and social issues

ROI Impact of Negative Investments on Wellbeing

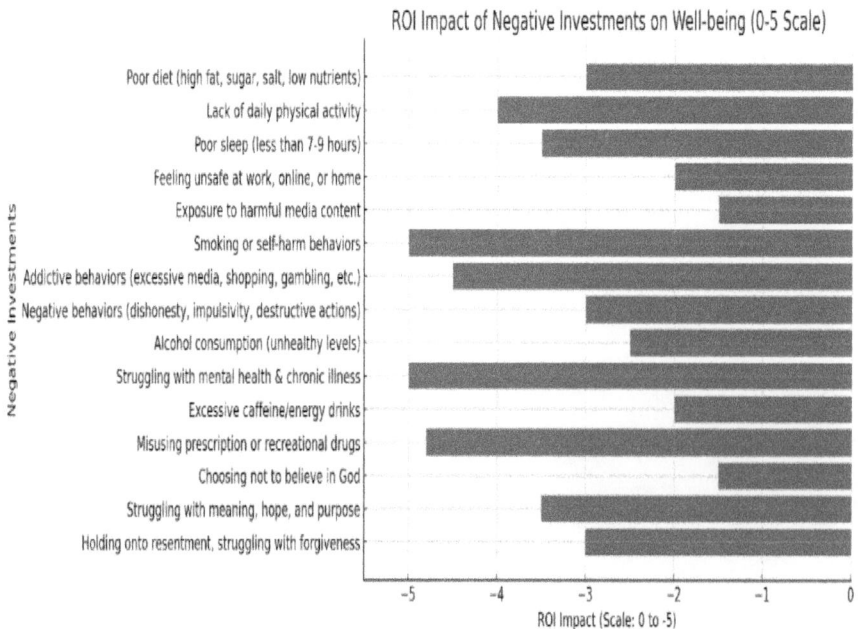

ROI Impact of Negative Investments on Well-being (0-5 Scale)

Negative Investments

The above visual representation is clear: negative investments produce a negative effect on our wellbeing. The question is: what is the impact and how significant is that impact on our life?

ROI Analysis of Positive & Negative Human Bank Investments

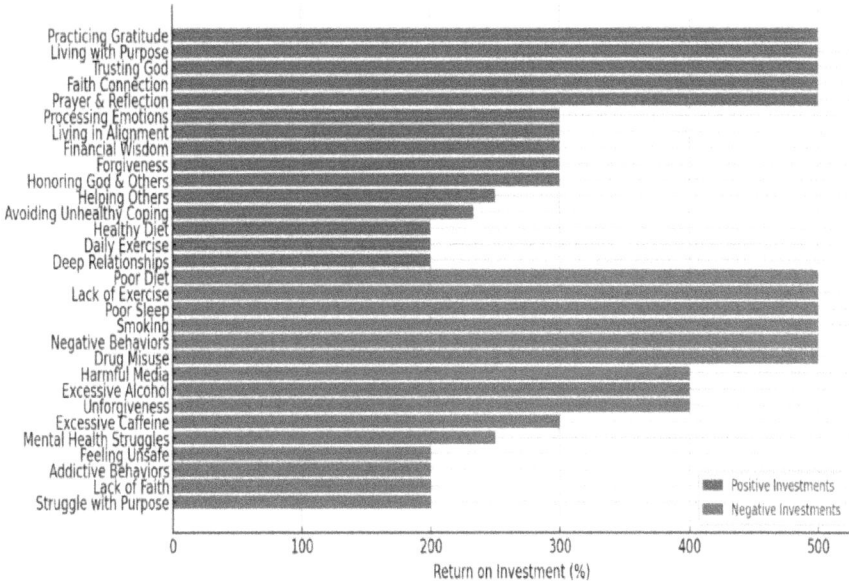

This chart shows two things:

- That returns on positive investments are positive.
- That returns on negative investments are negative.

In other words, if the investment is not positive, the return will not be, either.

I would like to highlight that point. Not making investments produces a negative return. Why? Because we are not investing into our wellbeing or Human Bank what it needs. This means it does not have adequate supply of Human Bank Currency to trade, so our Human Bank is in **loss**.

Can we take a moment to imagine the compounding impact on our life if we're making one, two, three, or even more negative investments?

Michael J. Smith

The Liability

Human Bank™ Liability - Definition

A negative investment, behaviour, or decision that creates a debt or burden within a person's Human Bank. Collective liabilities deplete Human Bank Currency across the five Human Banks and reduce a person's overall wellbeing and capacity to invest positively.

Unfortunately, when we are in a state of loss, we can create debt and liability in our Human Bank. To make up for the deficit, we sometimes seek other ways to pay our debt or to compensate for our lack of true Human Bank Currency. This is where people look for alternative ways to get by each day.

Human Bank™ Counterfeit/Foreign Currency

What happens when we are in the state of loss/bankruptcy in our Human Bank Currency? We turn to alternative sources of supply called **Counterfeit Currency**. We are familiar with this term from Chapter 4, and that it is an inferior substitute for real Human Bank Currency. Let's take a look at some counterfeit currencies that people use to supplement the deficit of Human Bank Currency:

Inferior substitutes for the Human Bank Currencies - external behaviours or influences that mimic value but ultimately deplete wellbeing.

Imitations of true Human Bank™ Currency that offer short-term stimulation but ultimately drain wellbeing. These external behaviours or influences may appear to provide Energy, Joy, Love, Peace, or Freedom—but result in depletion, disconnection, and long-term harm.

Human Bank™	Human Bank™ Currency	Counterfeit Substitute
Physical Bank	Energy	Stimulants (e.g., caffeine, sugar, drugs)
Emotional Bank	Joy	Pleasure & Entertainment (e.g., escapism, social media)

Human Bank™	Human Bank™ Currency	Counterfeit Substitute
Relational Bank	Love	Pornography (false intimacy)
Mental Bank	Peace	Substance Use (e.g., alcohol, sedatives)
Soul Bank	Freedom	Addiction (bondage disguised as liberty)

I would like to say these Counterfeit currencies have a varying serious significance on our wellbeing in how many Counterfeit currencies we invest and for how long.

If you take an apple from an apple tree, it will always be an apple that replaces it. However, if the tree is poisoned, it will produce bad fruit. In the same way, if we poison our body by putting bad things into it, we will produce bad fruit. But if we invest positively into our bodies, nourishing it with what we need, we will produce good fruit.

Counterfeit currency could also be considered **foreign currency**. The dictionary definition of foreign is "strange or unfamiliar"; if we invest into our Human Bank currency that is strange and unfamiliar, an inferior substitute for true currency, the return on investment will be the same. It is not the currency that a Human Banks is designed for, and thus it does not return a profitable outcome.

Spending counterfeit or foreign currencies represent our attempts to compensate for a shortage of Human Bank Currency. It is often a short-term strategy to get by, to make it through the day. Sadly, as it is a short-term fix, so are the outcomes. Foreign or counterfeit currency is not what the Human Bank needs; as it requires Human Bank Currency; the deficit remains. In a sense, energy, joy, peace, love and freedom are being denied to us or even being stolen from us.

Chapter 11: The Human Bank™ Diminishing Return

The Law of Human Bank™ Diminishing Return

"The law of diminishing marginal returns is a theory in economics that predicts that after some optimal level of capacity is reached, adding an additional factor of production will actually result in smaller increases in output."[19]

Let's define the Human Bank™ Law of Diminishing Return:

Human Bank™ Law of Diminishing Return - Definition

A principle stating that as we use our Human Bank Currency, its return begins to diminish. When one area of Human Bank Currency (e.g., Energy, Joy, Love, Peace, or Freedom) starts to decline, it negatively impacts the others because all five Human Banks are interconnected. As one depletes, the return on investment in other areas also diminishes, reducing overall wellbeing, capacity, potential and the profitability of the Human Bank™.

This is a powerful concept and one we need to grasp if we are to truly understand how our Human Bank works. All out five Human Banks are interrelated. In Chapter 6, Supply and Demand, we saw that our resources are finite, not infinite. We only have so much Human Bank Currency for each day, therefore and we need to spend and invest it wisely. When our Human Bank currencies diminish, so does our productivity, wellbeing and profitability.

"Many studies, including research from the International Labour Organisation, demonstrate that extending working hours beyond a certain point leads to a drop in productivity per hour worked, indicating diminishing returns to labour due to fatigue and decreased focus."[21]

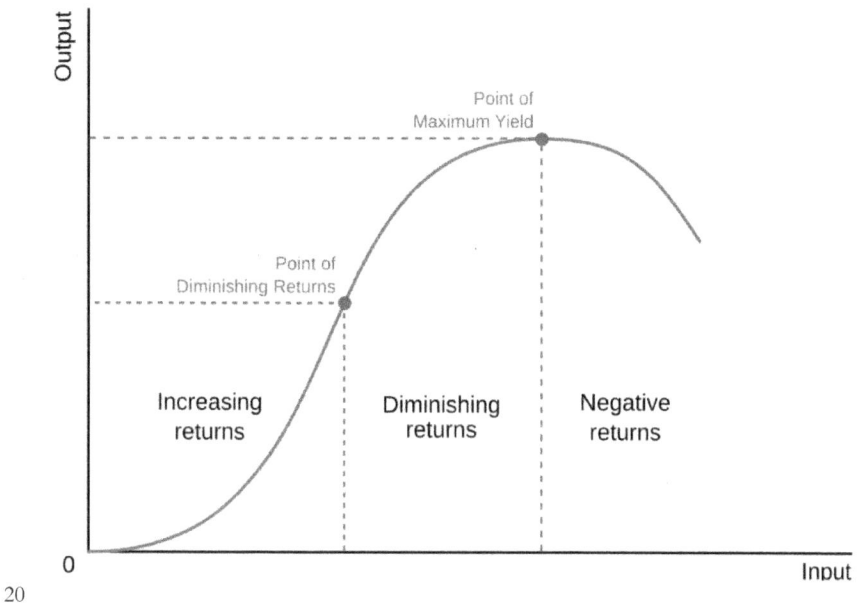

The Human Bank law of diminishing return means that when our Human Bank Currency diminishes so does our whole-life wellbeing and the profitability of our Human Bank. Consider that increased working hours can result in productivity decline:

Studies show the correlation between the increase of employee hours worked (inputs) results in the decrease of physical capacity, capability, productivity (outputs) as the length of time increases.

Interestingly, as time increases, productivity decreases to downward curve. Why is that? There are five factors involved. Let's call them our Human Bank Currency or production outputs:

- Physical Currency Output
- Emotional Currency Output
- Relational Currency Output
- Mental Currency Output
- Soul Currency Output

All five outputs are in operation in our daily working life. These outputs vary throughout our day. Let's assume at the start of the day we are at our optimal level. We've just slept, resting our bodies our minds, we consumed breakfast, perhaps had a coffee, all of which are inputs for a day of productivity.

At around mid-morning our energy and focus starts to diminish and we look for a morning snack and an excuse to get up and go for a walk. There is a slow decline from lunch time, and by mid-afternoon we are struggling to focus. By 5 p.m. our capacity is well and truly diminished after expending physical and mental energy.

We have diminished our production outputs. Our energy, joy, love, peace and freedom have all been spent achieving the optimal level of productive output. There is nothing left in our Human Bank. Then, the manager asks if we can work back a few hours to finish the project.

Our first thought is usually, *I just want to go home and rest.* But the money and the consequences of saying no is motivation enough to agree to work back. We buckle up for the next two hours.

The reality is we don't have the output necessary to continue producing at the same level of efficiency. Even though we stayed an extra two hours (which could equate to 25% of a normal working day) our actual output is significantly diminished. We find ourselves tired and distracted, struggling to focus, and end up being non-productive and frustrated for two hours. In this scenario we are experiencing Diminishing Return on our investment, being left more unproductive, drained and frustrated when you still have other personal things to attend to tonight.

You can see how if this cycle is repeated day after day, it depletes all our productive outputs, our physical emotional relational mental and soul currency, which has a significant impact on our Human Bank, productivity and overall wellbeing.

I can relate to this in my own life. Although the concepts have been with me for 20-plus years, it was not until 2025 that I actually committed to writing *Human Bank*. This led me to dedicate two months to focusing on writing fulltime. Putting a line in the sand and setting a release date meant that I had a fixed number of hours to complete the writing of the book. I needed the maximum amount of time I could to invest into achieving this deadline.

In reality, this meant working day and night in various ways on various things. Even though I had the Human Bank concept and understood how to maintain sustainable wellbeing productively and efficiently, I was experiencing diminishing returns; my night focus wasn't there, my clarity wasn't there, and all these things impacted my motivation, capability, and capacity. I was pushing beyond the Human Bank resources I had, physically, emotionally, relationally, mentally, and spiritually. I was pouring out everything one day, then feeling drained the next. I was in a place of deficit.

There wasn't some magical reset button that brought me back to 100% capacity overnight, but I increased my positive investments. I went for walks, I prayed, reflected, and rested.

I came back, got my breakfast, had my chai tea, and got ready to start the day. But you know, the sharpness wasn't there—the boost, the get-up-and-go, the vitality, the energy—it was lagging from the deficit the day before. I lacked what I needed for the day; I may have been operating at 50% of my productive potential.

We have all been there before. We need energy to get us across the line. We turn to high-energy snacks (code for high-sugar snacks), caffeine, or anything that can give us an energy boost and makes us feel better emotionally. This cycle continues, day after day.

When we continuously operate above our Human Bank Currency capacity, productivity and clarity decreases over the long term. I had to adjust my health and work schedule to bring it back into a sustainable range where I have the Human Bank Currency resources to meet daily demands, to hit that optimal level of demand and supply for the most efficient and sustainable output. At the same time, I am also investing positively back into myself so that I have the human capital resources in my Human Bank.

Organisational Management of Human Bank Currency Resources

This is the crux of the matter; what are the demands on the Human Bank Currencies (HBC) of organisations, management and their team? This is where demand meets supply. Consider:

- Does your team have the Human Bank Currency for their daily role?
- Is your team in profit in their Human Bank?
- Is your team in loss in their Human Bank?

You may not know the answer to these questions, but you will see it reflected in the performance and culture of your team.

How we manage our HBC, the demands we place on our team, and their ability to supply that demand is critical. It comes down to a lot of factors for an organisation: values, culture, strategic objectives, and the push-pull factors from stakeholders, the board, clients, and customers, all driving to extract the maximum output of human capital for maximum gain. The responsibility of balancing these demands ultimately rests with management and ourselves.

You may have heard the term "Social Responsibility" proclaimed in organisations. I would like to introduce a new term for the workplace: **"Wellbeing Responsibility"**. It is exactly what it suggests: corporations, organisations, and businesses taking responsibility for employee wellbeing. This encompasses both the demands and expectations of organisations and the wellbeing capacity of employees to supply that demand. If an organisation's demand exceeds the supply (wellbeing capacity) of its workforce, then disparity arises.

Fractional Reserve Lending Principle

This is a banking system in which banks are required to keep only a fraction of their deposits as reserves while they lend out the rest to borrowers. Banks do not lend out all the currency and money they have; they keep a portion – a buffer of it in case it is needed

Organisations need to adopt the Fractional Reserve Wellbeing Principle. This means organisations do not exhaust all their Human Bank Currency but instead keep reserves so that the collective Organisational Human Bank remains profitable— able to meet its future withdrawals.

If, however, an organisation decides to maximise gain and output, expending all its Human Bank Currency each day, **it will no longer be able to meet future Human Bank Currency demands** and will be trading insolvent in its collective Human Bank.

Let's use a running analogy; if we choose to sprint as fast as we can, we will only be able to run for a short period of time. On the other hand, if we run at a slower, sustainable pace, we will be able to run for a longer period of time. This conserves energy for the distance required.

The same theory applies to the supply of Human Bank Currency. If we demand that our employees all be sprinters and expend all their currency in a day, engaging in short, intense bursts, their Human Bank Currency resources will be depleted quickly.

Human Bank Diminishing Return

However, if we adopt the marathon runner approach—demanding small, sustainable quantities of Human Bank Currency over a longer period of time—the chances of both ourselves and our teams meeting that demand will increase exponentially, ensuring the sustainability of the organisation's collective Human Bank. This results in fewer diminishing returns.

Scarcity of Human Bank Currency will lead to lower production outputs. We need Human Bank Currency for production.

That being said, Human Bank Currency (HBC) resources are not just commodities to be traded, they must also be replenished in order to maintain sustainable supply to meet future demand. It is the responsibility of the individual employee to supply adequate Human Bank Currency and the responsibility of management not to over demand Human Bank Currency – this equals efficiency.

Under supply of HBC and over demand of HBC equals Human Bank failure– organisation stress. This happens when organisations, yielding to the tyranny of the urgent, sacrifice employee wellbeing on the altar of profit. This will clearly be seen in the bottom line and staff turnover, absenteeism, presenteeism, sick leave, stress leave and workers compensation claims. Consider that:

- Tired employees make unhappy employees.

- Unhappy employees are unproductive.

- Unproductive employees are counter-productive.

The Economic Cost of Poor Employee Wellbeing

Poor employee wellbeing has significant economic costs for organisations, impacting productivity, efficiency, engagement, and overall financial performance. Below are the key economic costs associated with poor wellbeing in the workplace:

1. Reduced Productivity & Performance

- Lower Output: Employees with poor wellbeing (physical, mental, emotional) struggle to maintain focus, efficiency, and performance, leading to decreased productivity.
- Presenteeism: Employees show up to work but underperform due to stress, burnout, or health issues, costing organisations 10 times more than absenteeism.
- Estimated Cost: Poor productivity due to wellbeing issues costs companies $1,500-$3,000 per employee annually (World Economic Forum).

2. Increased Absenteeism

- Health-Related Absences: Unhealthy employees take more sick days, on average, 50% more than healthier colleagues (Harvard Business Review).
Estimated Cost: Unscheduled absences cost businesses $2,660 per employee per year (Gallup).

3. Higher Employee Turnover & Recruitment Costs

- The cost of replacing an individual employee can range from one-half to two times the employee's annual salary— and that's a conservative estimate (Gallup).

4. Increased Healthcare & Insurance Costs

- Estimated Cost: Organisations spend $1,685 per employee, per year on healthcare due to stress-related illnesses (American Institute of Stress).

5. Poor Employee Engagement & Innovation

- Estimated Cost: Companies with low engagement levels see a 23% decrease in profitability (Gallup).

6. Workplace Accidents & Errors

- Higher Risk of Mistakes: Fatigue, stress, and poor concentration increase the likelihood of errors, misjudgements, and workplace accidents.

- Estimated Cost: Work-related stress accounts for $300 billion in global productivity losses annually (WHO).

7. Poor Customer Experience & Reputation Damage

- Estimated Cost: 80% of customers stop doing business with a company after a bad experience (PwC).

Key Statistics:

- The World Health Organization (WHO) estimates that mental health issues cost businesses around $1 trillion annually due to lost productivity.

- Gallup reports that employee burnout can cost businesses up to 15-20% of their total payroll due to voluntary turnover. 21

Note: References to *The Economic Cost of Poor Employee Wellbeing* can be found in the Footnote section of *The Human Bank™ References & Research.*

Conclusion: Organisations need to help their team effectively manage their Human Bank Currency so they have adequate Human Bank Currency to efficiently and effectively invest in their daily work demands.

If an organisation's goal is to demand all the Human Bank Currency or the wellbeing capacity of their team each day, **the result will most likely be the bankruptcy of their collective Human Bank**, resulting in staff turnover, disengagement, etc., as this is not sustainable and will deplete employee wellbeing. Organisations need to properly manage the demand and supply of Human Bank Currency to ensure they achieve optimal output and avoid diminishing return.

Chapter 12: The Human Bank™ Opportunity Cost

Opportunity Cost, "also known as alternative cost, is the value of the best option that's not chosen when making a decision. It's the potential benefits that are sacrificed by choosing one option over another."[27]

Human Bank™ Opportunity Cost - Definition

The Human Bank™ opportunity cost refers to the value of the wellbeing benefit lost when a person chooses one investment over another. It reflects the missed positive return that could have been gained if a more life-giving, restorative, or soul-aligned investment had been made. This impacts overall wellbeing across the five Human Banks.

The Human Bank™ Opportunity Cost is a powerful concept; it allows us to reflect on alternatives to our decisions, and most importantly, their potential consequences. In essence, it asks, "What am I forgoing or giving up by choosing this alternative?

It is a confronting question, one that forces us to consider:

- What are our wellbeing investments really costing us?

What physical, emotional, relational, mental, or soul wellbeing are we giving up by the actions and behaviours we chose? Sadly, we often turn in haste to the urgent or the exciting, pleasurable option that leads to some level of escape but sadly, the consequences are often left lagging in the initial gloss and appeal.

Consequence is the best friend of choice, but only if valued. What are the consequences of our actions on ourselves, others, our work, business, career, etc.? In the era of the "now" and "me" culture it seems people are less likely to consider the consequences of their actions, but the effects are real.

Previously, in the Demand and Supply chapter we saw some impacts up close. The impact of long work hours, high caffeine intake, high relational demands and poor diet day after day kept compounding, robbing the individual ultimately of their wellbeing, leading to negative coping methods.

Take a moment to pause and reflect:

- What is your current state of wellbeing?

- How are your wellbeing decisions made, and what are the consequences?

- How are these consequences impacting me, my family, friends, and colleagues?

- What would you like to be different?

Human Bank™ Opportunity Cost Model for 15 Negative Investments - Definition

The Human Bank Opportunity Cost Model reveals the evidence-based hidden cost of negative wellbeing investments. By choosing short-term comfort or unhealthy behaviours, individuals forfeit valuable Human Bank Currency. These lost returns such as increased Energy, Joy, Love, Peace, or Freedom represent the true opportunity cost of not making life-giving, Human Bank™ investments choices that benefit long-term wellbeing.

By engaging in short-term comforts or unhealthy behaviours, we forfeit long-term Human Bank Currency, weakening our overall wellbeing and our Human Bank. This model exposes the true cost of negative investments across the five Human Banks.

Below is an evidence-based analysis of the opportunity cost associated with each negative investment. For details on the research methodology and sources, refer to the *Human Bank™ References & Research* chapter.

Opportunity Cost Model for 15 Negative Human Bank™ Investments.

1. Physical Bank Wellbeing (Energy)

Negative Investment	Short-Term Comfort/ Convenience	Long-Term Opportunity Cost

Poor Nutrition (Unhealthy diet, high sugar, processed food)	Convenience, pleasure	Increased risk of Chronic, Disease, obesity, diabetes, cardiovascular disease
Lack of Exercise (Sedentary lifestyle, no daily movement)	Avoiding effort, saving time	Increased risk of Chronic, Weight gain, muscle loss, increased risk of depression
Poor Sleep (Less than 7–9 hours)	More time for work/social life	Cognitive impairment, weakened immune system, increased stress

1. Emotional Bank Wellbeing (Joy)

Negative Investment	Short-Term Comfort/ Convenience	Long-Term Opportunity Cost
Feeling Unsafe (Workplace, home, online)	Avoiding confrontation	Chronic stress, PTSD, social withdrawal
Exposure to Negative/Harmful Media (Violent, toxic, or fear-inducing content)	Entertainment, escapism	Increased anxiety, fear, emotional instability, aggression
Smoking & Substance Use (Nicotine, excessive drinking, drugs)	Temporary relaxation, stress relief	Addiction, reduced life expectancy, financial loss

2. Relational Bank Wellbeing (Love)

Negative Investment	Short-Term Comfort/ Convenience	Long-Term Opportunity Cost
Addictive Behaviours (Gaming, social media, gambling, excessive shopping)	Dopamine boost, instant gratification	Poor relationships, social isolation, financial issues

| Negative Behaviours (Dishonesty, impulsivity, destructive habits) | Short-term personal gain | Loss of trust, broken relationships, job instability |
| Excessive Alcohol Consumption (Four+ drinks daily) | Social bonding, stress relief | Liver damage, poor decision-making, career and family issues |

3. Mental Bank Wellbeing (Peace)

Negative Investment	Short-Term Comfort Convenience	Long-Term Opportunity Cost
Mental Health Struggles (Anxiety, depression, negative thoughts)	Avoiding therapy/treatment	Reduced cognitive function, lower career progression
Excessive Caffeine or Energy Drinks	Quick energy boost	Increased anxiety, heart palpitations, poor sleep
Drug Misuse (Recreational or prescription abuse)	Temporary escape, euphoria	Addiction, job loss, cognitive decline

5. Soul Bank Wellbeing (Freedom)

Negative Investment	Short-Term Comfort/ Convenience	Long-Term Opportunity Cost
Choosing Not to Believe in God	Sense of independence	Loss of meaning, lower resilience to life challenges
Lack of Meaning, Hope, or Purpose	Avoiding deep reflection	Increased risk of depression, lack of motivation

Holding Onto Resentment & Unforgiveness	Feeling justified, avoiding vulnerability	Higher stress, heart disease, social disconnection

Key Insights from the Opportunity Cost Model:

1. Failing to invest in positive wellbeing leads to long-term deficits. Poor physical and mental wellbeing leads to higher healthcare costs, reduced productivity, and increased stress.
2. Opportunity Cost = Missed wellbeing returns. Every time a positive wellbeing investment is neglected, there is a compounding negative effect in health, relationships, emotional stability, and life satisfaction.
3. Prioritising wellbeing is a long-term strategy. Investing in wellbeing is not just about short-term gains but about building resilience, increasing Human Bank Currency, and ensuring sustainable growth.
4. Short-term gains are illusions. Many negative investments provide instant gratification (e.g., food, alcohol, entertainment) but lead to long-term depletion in energy, productivity, health, and relationships and our Human Bank.
5. Lost potential multiplies over time. Each missed opportunity for positive investment results in cumulative losses. Over time, this leads to a compounded decline in Human Bank Currency and wellbeing.
6. Breaking the cycle requires awareness. Understanding opportunity costs allows individuals to make more conscious choices, shifting our focus from short-term comfort to long-term wellbeing.

Summary

The Human Bank operates like an economic system: if you fail to invest into your wellbeing, you incur long-term losses in health, productivity, and fulfilment. The opportunity cost of neglecting wellbeing isn't just short-term inconvenience, but long-term depletion of Human Bank Currency and loss of days spent with health and wellbeing.

Key Question: Are your daily investments building long-term wealth in your Human Bank, or are they trading short-term comfort for long-term decline?

Human Bank™ Opportunity Cost Model for 15 Positive Investments

The Human Bank™ Opportunity Cost Model reveals the evidence-based gains unlocked through positive wellbeing investments. By choosing life-giving, restorative actions over short-term comfort or unhealthy behaviours, individuals secure valuable Human Bank™ Currency. These returns — such as increased Energy, Joy, Love, Peace, and Freedom — represent the long-term rewards of making wise, intentional choices that build lasting Human Bank™ wellbeing.

Opportunity Cost Model for 15 Positive Human Bank™ Investments.

1. Physical Bank Wellbeing (Energy)

Positive Investment	Immediate Benefit	Opportunity Cost of Not Investing
Eating a Healthy & Nutritious Diet	Increased energy, improved digestion	Higher risk of chronic illness, obesity, heart disease
Daily Exercise (30-60 mins)	Cardiovascular health, reduced stress	Increased risk of obesity, diabetes, anxiety, and depression
Avoiding Unhealthy Coping Mechanisms	Emotional stability, long-term resilience	Increased reliance on unhealthy habits, decreased emotional regulation

2. Emotional Bank Wellbeing (Joy)

Positive Investment	Immediate Benefit	Opportunity Cost of Not Investing
Processing Emotions & Releasing Resentment	Emotional clarity, reduced stress	Increased anxiety, emotional outbursts, mental exhaustion
Living in Alignment with True Self	Higher self-esteem, purpose	Increased stress, identity struggles, dissatisfaction

Michael J. Smith

	Increased happiness, reduced negativity	Higher stress, lower life satisfaction, increased depressive symptoms
Expressing Gratitude Daily		

3. Relational Bank Wellbeing (Love)

Positive Investment	Immediate Benefit	Opportunity Cost of Not Investing
Helping & Supporting Others	Increased sense of purpose, deeper relationships	Social disconnection, loneliness, reduced life satisfaction
Cultivating Deep, Authentic Relationships	Emotional security, support network	Increased risk of isolation, higher stress, lower life expectancy
Managing Finances Wisely, Avoiding Debt	Reduced stress, financial security	Increased anxiety, financial struggles, limited future opportunities

4. Mental Bank Wellbeing (Peace)

Positive Investment	Immediate Benefit	Opportunity Cost of Not Investing
Practising Forgiveness	Reduced stress, emotional freedom	Higher stress, resentment, increased risk of heart disease
Living with Meaning & Purpose	Increased motivation, fulfilment	Depression, lack of direction, decreased motivation
Trusting in God & Letting Go of Worry	Emotional resilience, inner peace	Increased anxiety, fear, chronic stress

5. Soul Bank (Freedom)

Positive Investment	Immediate Benefit	Opportunity Cost of Not Investing

Connecting with God - Faith for Peace & Hope	Increased emotional stability, hope	Increased risk of depression, anxiety, and stress
Loving & Honouring God & Others	Sense of fulfilment, deeper relationships	Increased loneliness, dissatisfaction, moral struggles
Dedicating Time to Prayer & Reflection	Emotional clarity, lower stress	Higher levels of anxiety, lack of focus, decision fatigue

Key Insights from the Opportunity Cost Model

1. Negative investments have cumulative costs. The longer negative habits persist, the greater the opportunity cost in health, productivity, relationships, and happiness.
2. Wellbeing decline leads to economic loss. Poor wellbeing translates to increased medical costs, absenteeism, and lost productivity (WHO, 2021).
3. Shifting to positive investments yields higher returns. Investing in physical, emotional, relational, mental, and spiritual wellbeing creates compounded benefits over time.

Comparative Wellbeing Investment Analysis

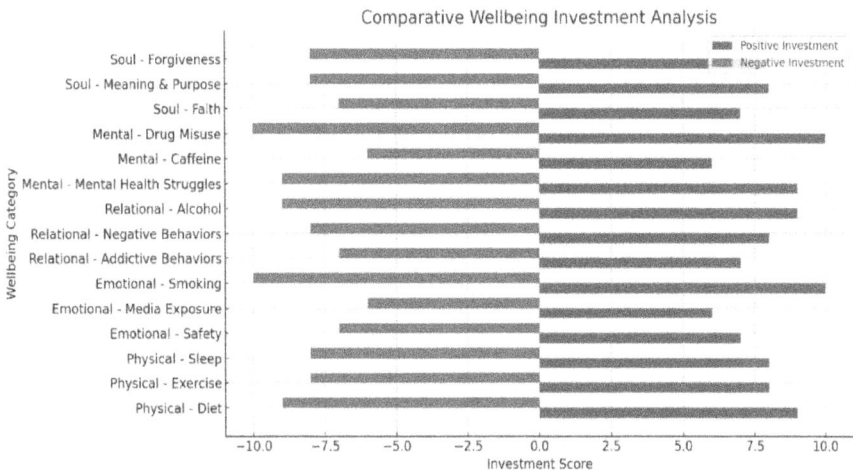

Comparative Wellbeing Investment Analysis

Every negative investment comes with a trade-off. The more we neglect wellbeing, the more future opportunities for fulfillment, energy, and success are sacrificed. Recognising and adjusting investments in Human Bank Currencies is the key to reversing long-term deficits and achieving sustainable wellbeing making the most out of life's opportunities. Life is for living, not for lost opportunities!

In conclusion

We need to be confronted with the potential reality of our wellbeing investment decisions and what we are forgoing by choosing those investment options. What is it costing us? What is it robbing from our wellbeing by not investing for positive and beneficial wellbeing returns?

When, we look at the opportunity cost of negative investments, it is very confronting. They are real-life impacts that you and I can experience. We could be trading our opportunity for physical, emotional, relational, mental or soul wellbeing for short-term feelings of satisfaction. Sadly, we often do not consider the consequences and their impact on our life and wellbeing. It is critical that we actually consider our choices and their short- and long-term cost on our Human Bank. It is important to know what is being stolen from our life. How our decisions are stealing our health and wellbeing and causing long-term consequences like chronic illness, disease, mental health challenges, anxiety, depression, and hopelessness. These all can be debilitating and life controlling.

We need to bring awareness to investments that improve our wellbeing, enabling us to truly prosper in life.

Organisational Opportunity Cost: The Human Bank™

Let's look at what organisations lose by neglecting wellbeing, and what they gain by investing in it. If the employee's Human Bank is bankrupt, the organisation's Human Bank is also bankrupt, and that results in huge financial and non-financial opportunity costs.

Organisational Opportunity Cost: The Human Bank™ Breakdown

Human Bank Area	If You Don't Invest (Costs)	If You Do Invest (Benefits)
Physical Bank (Energy)	↑ Absenteeism due to illness & fatigue, ↑ Health insurance costs, ↓ Productivity	↓ Sick leave, ↑ Energy & stamina, ↑ Operational output
Emotional Bank (Joy)	↓ Morale, ↑ Conflict, ↓ Engagement, ↑ Mental health claims	↑ Positivity, ↑ Team cohesion, ↑ Resilience under pressure
Relational Bank (Love)	Poor communication, ↑ Staff turnover, Toxic culture, ↓ Collaboration	Stronger team bonds, ↑ Retention, Better leadership & mentoring
Mental Bank (Peace)	↑ Stress leave, ↑ Mistakes/errors, ↓ Innovation, ↑ Burnout risk	↑ Focus, Better decision-making, ↑ Creativity & problem-solving
Soul Bank (Freedom)	↑ Meaninglessness, ↓ Job satisfaction, ↑ Quiet quitting, ↓ Values alignment	↑ Purpose-driven work, ↑ Loyalty, ↑ Initiative, ↓ Turnover

Key Insights:

If an organisation causes harm to the health and wellbeing of their employees, they won't be productive for very long. The opportunity cost of neglecting wellbeing is high. Lost productivity, staff turnover, health costs, poor morale, reputational damage, and burnout are expensive, financially and culturally. **The opportunity cost of ignoring employee wellbeing is more than lost productivity: it's lost innovation, loyalty, culture and long-term business viability.**

The Purpose of the Human Bank Model

In a competitive market where skilled and experienced labour is in short supply, the main recourse for poor employee wellbeing is to leave. Sustainable employee wellbeing leads to a sustainable labour market and productive output. Healthy and happy employees far outweigh the opportunity cost of unhappy and unhealthy employees.

Human Bank Opportunity Cost is all about not forgoing the benefits of employees having health and prosperous Human Bank. It is designed to help both organisations and their employees; it's a win for all. The R.O.I. in the Human Bank™ model is measurable and transformative, resulting in:

- Healthier people

- Stronger teams

- Better business outcomes

- A thriving, resilient, purpose-driven organisation.

Organisations that value and care for their employees will likely result in employees valuing and caring for the organisation.

Chapter 13: The Human Bank™ Cost Benefit

In the previous chapter we explored the cost of wellbeing opportunities missed because of the decisions we make. Having examined the potential impacts of missed opportunities on our Human Bank, we will now shift our attention to the Costs and Benefits of our Human Bank™ Investments.

Human Bank™ Cost Benefit Analysis (HBCBA) - Definition

Human Bank Cost-Benefit refers to the process of evaluating the personal wellbeing costs and potential benefits of a Human Bank™ investment—whether Physical, Emotional, Relational, Mental, or Soul-based. It helps determine whether a choice results in a positive return (profit) or a negative return (loss) to the five Human Banks.

Once again, we will refer to the 15 Positive and 15 Negative Human Bank™ Investments introduced in Chapter 5. This will help you better understand what each daily investment costs you and the benefits it brings to your wellbeing. The following Human Bank™ Cost-Benefit Analysis (CBA) outlines these investments, supported by relevant evidence.

This model supports wiser investment decisions by weighing:

Benefits gained - Energy, Joy, Love, Peace, Freedom
Costs incurred - Burnout, Stress, Depletion, Regret, Addiction.

Key Questions:

- What is your wellbeing costing you?
- Is the cost of your daily investments greater than the benefits?

Human Bank™ Positive Investment Cost-Benefit Analysis

Physical Bank:

1. **Daily consumption of a healthy and nutritious diet (rich in fruits & vegetables, low in fat, salt, sugar):**
    Benefits:
    -   Enhanced physical health and reduced risk of chronic diseases.
    -   Improved energy levels.

    Costs:
    -   Time of shopping, preparation, cooking.
    -   Potential higher cost of healthy foods.

2. **Daily engaging in exercise (30-60 mins daily):**
    Benefits:
    -   Improved strength and cardiovascular health and reduced risk of chronic diseases.
    -   Enhanced mood, outlook and mental health.

    Costs:
    -   Time commitment.
    -   Possible cost for clothing, equipment or gym membership.

3. **Daily exercising self-control to avoid unhealthy coping mechanisms (e.g., excessive media, eating, drinking, substance use):**
    Benefits:
    -   Improved mental clarity, greater freedom and emotional health.
    -   Enhanced physical, emotional, relational, mental and soul wellbeing.

    Costs:
    -   Physical, emotional. mental currency to develop healthier habits.
    -   Forgoing temporary pleasures.

Emotional Bank:

1. **Daily processing feelings, releasing anger, and letting go of bitterness:**
    Benefits:
    -   Emotional freedom and reduced stress, anger, and bitterness levels.
    -   Improved relationships, experience of love and connection.

Costs:
- Emotional, relational soul energy processing upset.
- Time invested in communication, conflict resolution or self-reflection.

2. **Daily living in alignment with authentic 'True' self; values, beliefs, passions, and purpose:**
   Benefits:
   - Increased life meaning and fulfillment.
   - Clarity and direction in decision-making.
   Costs:
   - Potential social and relationship conflicts and cost with social expectations.
   - Sacrifice of other alternatives.

3. **Daily expressing gratitude, recognising contentment with life:**
   Benefits:
   - Enhanced joy, freedom and optimism.
   - Improved relationships and peace.
   Costs:
   - Minimal time investment.

Relational Bank:
1. **Daily offering help and support to those in need:**
   Benefits:
   - Strengthened relationships, sense of community and connection.
   - Personal fulfillment - investing into your own Human bank.
   Costs:
   - Time and resources spent.

2. **Daily cultivating deep, authentic relationships with supportive individuals:**
   Benefits:
   - Strengthened self-worth, identity, sense of belonging.
   - Enhanced physical, emotional, relational, mental and soul wellbeing.
   Costs:

- Time, physical, emotional, relational and mental investment.

3. **Daily managing finances wisely, ensuring enough money for essentials and avoiding debt:**
   Benefits:
   - Financial security and reduced stress.
   - Enhanced overall peace and contentment.
   - Ability to invest in future opportunities.

   Costs:
   - Time spent budgeting.
   - Potential sacrifices, saying "No".

Mental Bank:

1. **Daily practicing forgiveness, for others and oneself:**
   Benefits:
   - Improved emotional, mental, soul freedom.
   - Emotional liberation and improved.
   - Enhanced relationships, inner peace and mental health.

   Costs:
   - Emotional effort.
   - Overcoming personal grievances.

2. **Daily living with a sense of meaning and purpose guiding actions:**
   Benefits:
   - Improved decision making and mental clarity.
   - Enhanced motivation and determination.
   - Overall life satisfaction and flourishing of the Human Bank.

   Costs:
   - Time spent in self-reflection and preparation.
   - Potential lifestyle and behavioural changes.

3. **Daily trusting in God with things beyond control:**
   Benefits:
   - Enhanced overall physical, emotional, relational, mental and soul wellbeing.
   - Increased inner peace and reduced anxiety.

- Sense of spiritual connection and freedom.
- Invests in all the Human Banks.

Costs:

- Personal time dedicated to talking with God - prayer.

Soul Bank:

1. **Daily experiencing a connection to faith in God, bringing love, peace, and hope:**
   Benefits:
   - Flourishing soul, overflowing with life and vitality.
   - Experiencing deep inner peace, freedom and belonging.

   Costs:
   - Time and commitment to faith-based activities and spiritual practices; abiding in God, with His love, peace and hope.

2. **Daily living to love and honour God and others with actions:**
   Benefits:
   - Cultivates deep connection with God and others.
   - Enhances overall freedom.
   - Personal meaning, fulfillment and moral alignment.

   Costs:
   - Self-sacrifice.
   - Effort and energy in practicing love and service.

3. **Daily dedicating time to prayer and personal Bible reading:**
   Benefits:
   - Improved clarity, peace of mind and reducing stress.
   - Connect with God and His love, peace and truth.
   - Enhancing overall wellbeing and flourishing of our Human Bank.

   Costs:
   - Time allocation for prayer and Bible reading.
   - Need a quiet place.
   - Sacrificing time for other things.

Human Bank™ Negative Investment Cost-Benefit Analysis

Physical Bank:

1. **Poor Diet: Daily, I do not nourish my body with a balanced diet rich in fruits and vegetables while limiting unhealthy fats, salt, and sugar:**

   Costs:
   - Currency costs: energy, joy, love, peace and freedom, through:
   - Increases the risk of chronic diseases such as heart disease, stroke, and type 2 diabetes and other related health issues.
   - Affects overall life wellbeing and our Human Bank.

   Benefits:
   - Convenience and lower immediate food costs.

2. **Physical Inactivity: Daily, I do not engage in at least 30–60 minutes of physical activity to strengthen my body and improve my wellbeing:**

   Costs:
   - Currency costs: energy, joy, love, peace and freedom, through:
   - Decreased strength, poor circulation, weight gain, and increased stress.
   - Elevates the risk of noncommunicable diseases (NCDs) and other poor health outcomes.
   - Affects overall life wellbeing and Human Bank.

   Benefits:
   - More time available for other activities.

3. **Insufficient Sleep: Daily, I do not prioritise getting 7–9 hours of restful sleep to restore my energy and health:**

   Costs:
   - Currency costs - energy, joy, love, peace and freedom, through:
   - Fatigue, poor concentration, reduced immunity, and mental health struggles.
   - Negatively affects physical energy, emotional mood, relational stress, cognitive functions, and level of peace.
   - Increase stress and irritability.

   Benefits:
   - More waking hours for work or leisure.

Emotional Bank:

1. **Feeling Unsafe: Daily, I struggle to feel safe in the workplace, online, or at home:**

    Costs:
    -   Currency costs: energy, joy, love, peace and freedom, through:
    -   Ongoing stress, fear, and anxiety, affecting emotional security.
    -   Leads to decreased freedom, peace, limits choices, productivity, soul, emotional and mental health and quality of life overall.

    Benefits:
    -   May prompt greater security measures and caution.

2. **Exposure to Dark and Harmful Media: Daily, I expose myself to dark or harmful media, including violent content, coarse language, negativity, or sexualised material:**

    Costs:
    -   Currency costs: energy, joy, love, peace and freedom, through:
    -   Normalising violence and negative behaviours.
    -   Fosters negativity, reduces joy, and increases stress.
    -   May increase loss of freedom through anxiety, fear, stress and distorted perceptions of reality, sexualisation, violent behaviour.

    Benefits:
    -   Provides entertainment and escapism.

3. **Smoking: Daily, I engage in smoking, harming my body and long-term health:**

    Costs:
    -   Currency costs: energy, joy, love, peace and freedom, through:
    -   Loss of long-term health and causes addiction.
    -   Increases the risk of addiction, chronic respiratory illness and other health complications.
    -   Potentially reduces life expectancy.
    -   Affects overall life wellbeing and our Human Bank.

    Benefits:

- Short-term stress relief and social bonding.

Relational Bank:

1. **Engaging in Addictive Behaviours: Daily, I engage in addictive behaviours (e.g., excessive social media use, video gaming, online shopping, TV streaming, excessive working, compulsive internet use, pornography, gambling, smoking, drinking, or substance use) that feel out of my control:**

    Costs:
    - Currency costs: energy, joy, love, peace and freedom, through:
    - Loss of control, emotional detachment, and neglect of meaningful relationships.
    - Can lead to physical and psychological dependence.
    - Loss of personal freedom, choice and capacity.
    - Negatively impacts relationships and social interactions.

    Benefits:
    - Provides temporary pleasure or escape.

2. **Negative Behaviours: Daily, I exhibit negative behaviours such as dishonesty, impulsivity, or destructive words and actions that harm myself and others:**

    Costs:
    - Currency costs: energy, joy, love, peace and freedom, through:
    - Damaging trust, increasing conflicts, and isolating individuals from loved ones.
    - Leads to long-term relational destruction, reputational harm, disconnection.
    - Potentially lead to guilt, shame and regret.

    Benefits:
    - May offer short-term gains or advantages but ultimately cost i.e. getting away with lying, taking advantage of people.

3. **Excessive Alcohol Consumption: Daily, I drink alcohol, often in unhealthy amounts (four or more drinks):**

    Costs:
    - Currency costs: energy, joy, love, peace and freedom, through:

- Increased risk of long-term damage to health and relationships.
- Increases the risk of addiction and various health issues, including liver disease and cancer.
- Impairs judgment and coordination, can lead to accidents, injuries and destructive behaviours.
- Reduces freedom of choice and behaviour.

Benefits:
- Provides temporary escape, relaxation and social interaction.

Mental Bank:

1. **Struggling with Mental Health Issues: Daily, I struggle with mental health and with chronic illness challenges such as chronic pain, depression, fear, anxiety, or continual negative thoughts:**

   Costs:
   - Currency costs: energy, joy, love, peace and freedom, through:
   - Increased risks of depression, anxiety, and emotional distress.
   - Reduces quality of life, daily functioning and independence.
   - Increases the risk of social isolation, chronic diseases and substance abuse.
   - Decreases freedom, choice, capacity, and peace.

   Benefits:
   - May increase empathy towards others with similar struggles.

2. **Excessive Caffeine or Energy Drink Consumption: Daily, I consume excessive amounts (two or more) of caffeine or energy drinks, negatively impacting my health.**

   Costs:
   - Currency costs: energy, joy, love, peace and freedom, through:
   - Restlessness, poor sleep, and long-term health problems.
   - Negatively impacts sleep quality and cardiovascular health.
   - Can lead to dependence and increased anxiety.

Benefits:
- Provides temporary alertness and energy boost.

3. **Drug Misuse: Daily, I regularly misuse prescription or recreational drugs, affecting my wellbeing:**
   Costs:
   - Currency costs: energy, joy, love, peace and freedom, through:
   - Harming vital organs and increases the risk of overdose and death.
   - Leads to addiction and deteriorating mental health, freedom, and choice.
   - Reducing overall health, wellbeing, quality of life.
   - Can damage relationships, cause conflict and abuse.

   Benefits:
   - May offer temporary euphoria or escape from reality.

Soul Bank:

1. **Lack of Belief in God: Daily, each day, I choose not to believe in God:**
   Costs:
   - Currency costs: energy, joy, love, peace and freedom, through:
   - Spiritual emptiness, hopelessness, and moral confusion.
   - Enhanced stress, anxiety, meaninglessness.
   - Increasing lack of love, lack of peace, lack of joy, lack of freedom, and mental health challenges.

   Benefits:
   - Encourages self-reliance and personal responsibility.

2. **Struggling to Find Meaning or Purpose: Daily, I struggle to find meaning, hope, or purpose, leaving me feeling lost or unfulfilled:**
   Costs:
   - Currency costs: energy, joy, love, peace and freedom, through:
   - Increases feelings of depression, lack of motivation, and an inner void.
   - Increases the risk of depression and anxiety.
   - Leads to decreased motivation, identity and life satisfaction, self-worth.

Benefits:
- May prompt exploration and personal growth.

3. **Difficulty Forgiving: Daily, I find it difficult to forgive myself and others, holding onto resentment, hurt, and pain.**
   Costs:
   - Currency costs: energy, joy, love, peace and freedom, through:
   - Causes emotional baggage, bitterness, and prolonged suffering.
   - Fosters resentment, anger, bitterness, leading to chronic stress and health issues.
   - Damages relationships and social connections.
   - Increases conflict, relational breakdown, negative and destructive behaviour.
   - Can lead to negative coping methods.

Note: For the *Research Methodology Summary* and the *Human Bank™ Cost-Benefit Analysis (HBCBA) Framework* evidence and methodology, see the *Human Bank™ References & Research* section.

I hope this chapter, which explores the evidence-based costs and benefits of our wellbeing decisions, has provided both insight and motivation. May it inspire you to avoid the costly wellbeing investments that carry both short-term and long-term consequences impacting not only your personal wellbeing and Human Bank™ but also your financial health.

My encouragement to you is this:
Actively pursue positive wellbeing investments. The benefits both immediate and lasting can enrich your life for years to come.

Remember, the cost of negative investments can take years to undo.
Now is a great time to start.

I'm cheering you on!

Chapter 14: The Human Bank™ Investment Strategy

Human Bank™ Investment Strategy - Definition

An intentional wellbeing plan based on the 15 Positive and 15 Negative Human Bank Investments. Its goal is to increase life-giving positive investments that strengthen the five Human Banks - Physical, Emotional, Relational, Mental, and Soul while decreasing negative investments that deplete or damage them. This strategy helps individuals build long-term wellbeing, spiritual alignment, and a profitable return on life.

Well done! You've come this far now is the opportunity to start planning your Human Bank Investment Strategy.

Below are Positive and Negative investments that you can make. To begin, choose three Positive Investments to do and three Negative Investments to avoid. Seek to build these into your daily routine and belief system. Develop a strategy around how to do the positives and how to avoid the negatives.

Each day, each step, each investment is a step closer to improving your Human Bank your overall wellbeing.

Celebrate the little steps. Over time, they accumulate into a very big step forward.

Positive Human Bank™ Investments - Definition

The 15 Positive Investment actions that deposit life-giving value into the five Human Banks - Physical, Emotional, Relational, Mental, and Soul. These investments fill and prosper your Human Bank, and build long-term wellbeing.

Negative Human Bank™ Investments - Definition

The 15 Negative Investment actions that drain, deplete, or damage the five Human Banks - Physical, Emotional, Relational, Mental, and Soul. These actions withdraw value, diminish long-term wellbeing, and can lead to burnout and the eventual bankruptcy of your Human Bank.

Physical Human Bank™ Investment Strategy

Make Physical Bank Positive Investments:

- ✓ Daily, I eat a healthy and nutritious diet (high in fruit & vegetables and low in fat, salt, sugar).
- ✓ Daily, I experience exercise (30-60 mins).
- ✓ Daily, I have self-control to avoid unhealthy coping mechanisms (e.g., excessive eating, excessive drinking, avoidance, substance use, isolation, excessive screen time, media, or shopping) to deal with stress, anxiety, or negative emotions.

Avoid Physical Bank Negative Investments:

- ✗ Each day, I do not nourish my body with a balanced diet rich in fruits and vegetables while limiting unhealthy fats, salt, and sugar.
- ✗ Each day, I do not engage in at least 30–60 minutes of physical activity to strengthen my body and improve my well-being.
- ✗ Each day, I do not prioritise getting 7–9 hours of restful sleep to restore my energy and health.

Emotional Human Bank™ Investment Strategy

Make Emotional Bank Positive Investments:

- ✓ Each day, I heal emotional upset by processing my feelings, releasing anger, and letting go of bitterness and resentment.
- ✓ Each day, I live in alignment with my authentic 'True' self; my values, beliefs, passions, and purpose.
- ✓ Each day, I express gratitude, recognising that while I may not have everything I want or need, I am content with my life.

Avoid Emotional Bank Negative Investments:

- ✗ Each day, I struggle to feel safe in the workplace, online, or at home.
- ✗ Each day, I expose myself to dark or harmful media, including violent content, coarse language, negativity, or sexualised material.

✗ Each day, I engage in smoking, harming my body and long-term health.

Relational Human Bank™ Investment Strategy

Make Relational Bank Positive Investments:

✓ Each day, I offer help and support to those in need in my life.
✓ Each day, I cultivate deep, authentic relationships with people who uplift and support me.
✓ Each day, I have enough money for essentials and spend my money wisely, avoiding debt.

Avoid Relational Bank Negative Investments:

✗ Each day, I engage in addictive behaviours (e.g., excessive social media use, video gaming, online shopping, TV streaming, excessive working, compulsive internet use, pornography, gambling, smoking, drinking, or substance use) that feel out of my control.
✗ Each day, I exhibit negative behaviours such as dishonesty, impulsivity, or destructive words and actions that harm myself and others.
✗ Each day, I drink alcohol, often in unhealthy amounts (four or more drinks).

Mental Human Bank™ Investment Strategy

Make Mental Bank Positive Investments:

✓ Each day, I practice forgiveness, both for others and for myself.
✓ Each day, I live with a sense of meaning and purpose that guides my actions.
✓ Each day, I trust in God with things beyond my control.

Avoid Mental Bank Negative Investments:

✗ Each day, I struggle with mental health and with chronic illness challenges such as chronic pain, depression, fear, anxiety, or continual negative thoughts.

✘ Each day, I consume excessive amounts (two or more) of caffeine or energy drinks, negatively impacting my health.

✘ I regularly misuse prescription or recreational drugs, affecting my wellbeing.

Soul Human Bank™ Investment Strategy

Make Soul Bank Positive Investments:

✓ Each day, I experience a connection to my faith in God that brings me love, peace, and hope.

✓ Each day, I live to love and honour God and others with my actions.

✓ Each day, I dedicate time to prayer and personal reflection.

Avoid Soul Bank Negative Investments:

✘ Each day, I choose not to believe in God.

✘ Each day, I struggle to find meaning, hope, or purpose, leaving me feeling lost or unfulfilled.

✘ Each day, I find it difficult to forgive myself and others, holding onto resentment, hurt, and pain.

Be intentional about building these positive investments into your daily life. One by one, they will become routine and begin to build health and wellbeing. You will notice many of the negative investments will dissipate, and you will be empowered to reduce them with God's help.

Keep investing in life that is true life!

Chapter 15: The Central Bank of the Human Bank™

I now want to introduce the Central Bank of the Human Bank.

Central Bank of the Human Bank™ - Definition

The central governing system of a person's inner life—representing the soul as the seat of identity, decision-making, and spiritual alignment. Just as a central bank regulates currency in an economy, the soul guides values, priorities, and how Human Bank Currency is invested across the five Human Banks: Physical, Emotional, Relational, Mental, and Soul.

The Soul Bank functions as the Central Bank of the Human Bank, and our will serves as the Governor. It has often been said that our mind, will, and emotions are functions of the soul. This is why the Soul Bank acts as the regulatory centre, overseeing the investment and spending decisions within our Human Bank.

We will explore the soul more deeply in the next chapter.

There are amazing parallels between the Central Banks of the financial world and the Central Bank of the Human Bank. Here is a summary of the role of the Human Bank and Central Bank (HBCB), in which we will compare the role of Central Banks in the financial world to the Central Bank of our Human Bank:

National Central Bank vs. Human Bank Central Bank: A Comparison

#	National Central Bank	Human Bank Central Bank
1	Implements monetary policy; regulates money supply and interest rates to promote economic stability.	Regulates the supply of Human Bank Currency to the Human Banks, through decisions we make.

2	Issues currency; controls the issuance of national currency to ensure financial trust and stability.	Controls the issuing of Human Bank Currency, through will and actions, to maintain stability.
3	Regulates commercial banks; supervises financial institutions to maintain a safe and sound banking system.	Supervises the five Human Banks' deposits and withdrawals and governs investment decisions.
4	Manages foreign exchange & reserves; oversees exchange rates and maintains foreign currency reserves.	Processes foreign currency into the Human Bank, also referred to as Counterfeit Currency (any substitute currency that is not true Human Bank Currency).
5	Ensures financial stability; monitors risks, prevents banking crises, and supports economic growth.	Monitors risks, seeks to prevent crises, and supports the profitability of the Human Bank through self-regulation and self-protection mechanisms.

As you can see the Central Bank plays a critical role in governance, oversight, controlling, monitoring, managing and preventing risk to our Human Bank.

Like real-world financial banks, the Human Bank can be subject to crises, even bankruptcy. Just as demany banks experienced in the 2008 Financial Crisis, prompting many governments to intervene, attempting to regulate, monitor and control the monetary system.

The system can be overrun; it can be manipulated and exploited, as we saw the Financial Crisis, where borrowing and debt went beyond safe regulatory levels with debt that was unsustainable for the banks to manage or to repay. Banks collapsed in insolvency, no longer able to function.

The failure of the banks had a cascading effect which impacted millions of people, placing them in financial bankruptcy. This is much the same as the wellbeing crisis that we're seeing at the moment. It effects millions of people globally. Moreover, it impacts people's ability to be gainfully employed, to be healthy, productive contributors to society and achieve their goals and aspirations.

People are exhausted, stressed, depressed, anxious, fearful, struggling with mental illness and chronic illness, to name a few consequences. The wellbeing crisis has a ripple effect which impacts relationships, homes, families, workplace, communities and nations. People struggle through the effects of physical bankruptcy, emotional bankruptcy, relational bankruptcy, mental bankruptcy, and soul bankruptcy any way they can.

- Bankruptcy in the Physical Bank means people have no **Energy**

- Bankruptcy in the Emotional Bank means people do not have **Joy**

- Bankruptcy in the Relational Bank means people are lacking in **Love**

- Bankruptcy in the Mental Bank means people have no **Peace**

- Bankruptcy in the Soul Bank means people do not experience **Freedom**

These stresses can compound, causing the person to feel like they are free-falling spiralling into a vortex of hopelessness and despair.

When people aren't operating profitably or sustainably in their Human Bank there are significant flow-on effects to themselves and the nation, including higher healthcare cost and reduced productivity. Not to mention, increased social issues, relational conflict, substance use, stealing, negative behaviours, anger violence, and other crime.

This is the Global Wellbeing Crisis. The Human Banks of millions of people across the world are bankrupt. The Physical Bank, Emotional Bank, Relational Bank, Mental Bank and Soul Bank are empty; they have nothing left to give, experiencing burn out, stress, anxiety, personal and relational breakdown. The global wellbeing banking system is collapsing. We need to take drastic action to intervene to invest back into our Human Banks so we can operate effectively, providing us with the wellbeing we need daily.

How do we do that? There is no quick fix, but there is a solution to this wellbeing crisis. It begins with the individual, and returning them to a state of wellbeing. This not only has impacts in the individual's life, but in their family, community, and nation. It starts with good investing, and that needs to start today.

One thing that becomes clear is that the Soul Bank plays a significant role in our wellbeing, arguably more so than the other four Human Banks. It helps us to regulate deposits and withdrawals to and from our Human Banks. In doing so it fulfills the role of the Central Bank. As stated at the beginning of the chapter, every Central Bank has a Governor. That is the subject we will explore in the next chapter.

Chapter 16: The Soul and Conscience

As discussed in Chapter 15, the soul is central to the governance of the Human Bank. Consider this definition of the soul:

> **"The principle of life, feeling, thought, and action in humans**, regarded as a distinct entity separate from the body, and commonly held to be separable in existence from the body; the spiritual part of humans as distinct from the physical part."

The Soul Bank is the Central Bank of our Human Bank because it is the "the principle of life, feeling, thought, and action in humans." In other words, it is:

- **'The principle of life'** - our 'true self'; our identity, our purpose, the spiritual part of us.
- **'Feeling'** – emotions.
- **'Thought'** - beliefs and decisions.
- **'Action'** - acting on beliefs and decisions.

It would be reasonable to say this encompasses our core function: our thoughts, feelings and actions. They all emanate from our soul, the spiritual part of our being. In other words, the soul is our true self: our feelings, our thoughts, will and desires. It is where our decision and actions flow out of. This is why it seeks to regulate our investments.

When our soul is healthy it leads us into good actions and behaviours - positive investments. However, when our soul is not healthy, we make poor wellbeing decisions and actions - negative Human Bank investments, which produce negative returns.

At the core of our soul and our decision-making is our conscience. The dictionary defines conscience as:

> "the inner sense of what is right or wrong in one's conduct or motives, impelling one toward right action: to follow the dictates of conscience."

In other words, the conscience is the part of a person that judges how moral their own actions are and makes them feel guilty about bad things that they have done or things they feel responsible for. For example;

- A **guilty conscience**: "He's been so kind and generous towards me recently, I think he's got a guilty conscience" (= feels guilty).
- A **clear conscience**: "You didn't do anything wrong, you should have a clear conscience" (= not feel guilty).

Our conscience seeks to lead and guide us to right actions and behaviours. It also warns us against wrong and potentially damaging actions and behaviours. It does this by causing us to feel guilt, shame or remorse for considering or doing something bad. It is a function of our 'True self': our soul communicating through our conscience that what we did was right or wrong and may or may not have negative consequences. If we did the wrong thing, we experience a guilty conscience, similar to the example given above.

Further definitions of 'conscience':

- "Conscience reveals to us a moral law whose source cannot be found in the natural world... and must therefore come from something outside of it — a divine Lawgiver." – C. S. Lewis
- "Senses involving consciousness of morality or what is considered right." – C. S. Lewis
- The internal acknowledgement or recognition of the moral quality of one's motives and actions; the sense of right and wrong as regards things for which one is responsible; the faculty or principle which judges the moral quality of one's actions or motives." - Oxford English Dictionary 22

We are accountable to our conscience for our actions. There are consequences for our actions; wrong actions can take away our peace, our joy, and gives us guilt, shame, and can make us feel bad and unclean. If we ignore our conscience, we go against ourselves.

One last definition:

"(i) practical reasoning about moral matters, which, though fallible, must be obeyed (Aquinas); (ii) the understanding which distinguishes between right and wrong and between virtue and vice; (iii) an infallible, God-given guide of conduct." 22

It is critical that we seek to be led by the moral compass of our soul, allowing it to guide us in paths of life, love, truth and freedom.

"Let us draw near with a true heart in full assurance of faith, with our hearts sprinkled clean from an evil conscience and our bodies washed with pure water." Hebrews 10:22

Chapter 17: The Governor of the Human Bank™

We have looked at Central Banks, and their role and function in regulating the monetary and banking system. We have also referred to the role of the Central Bank Governor. The Governor is the chief executive responsible for overseeing and implementing monetary policies and managing the central bank's operations. They are the 'Chairperson' that leads the governing board of the bank, deciding strategies to help the Central Bank control, supply and regulate currency in the financial market to ensure a stable financial system that creates trust and market participation. The Governor can change, and is elected by the Governing Board. This chapter focuses on the concept of the Governor of the Human Bank, and its role.

Who is the Governor (of the Human Bank™)?

The Governor is your Will, the internal decision-making authority that regulates how Human Bank Currency is invested or withdrawn across the five Human Banks: Physical, Emotional, Relational, Mental, and Soul. The Governor can be influenced to override the inner moral conscience, our sense of right and wrong which is governed by the Central Bank of the Human Bank™: the Soul.

Let's define it further:

The Governor controls the supply of Human Bank Currency:

- Your **will** is the **Governor** of your **soul**.

- Your **soul** governs your **Central Bank**.

- Your **Central Bank** governs your **Human Banks**.

Your **Will** decides your actions and behaviours. In other words, you govern your Human Bank through your will, desires, passion, intellect, emotions, thoughts, and beliefs, which come from your soul.

What influences our will? Input. We receive input from our five senses: things we see, touch, taste, smell, and hear all get processed in the soul. These trigger thoughts and desires that seek to influence our will. Therefore, we act out our will, from those thoughts and desires.

This is why marketing and advertising can be so influential. It is the communication of information for goods and services that hope to foster desires in us for those products and services, thus activating our will to act on those desires by obtaining the product or service.

The soul is the seat of our decision-making process; we receive inputs, process those inputs as information and then our will is formed and a decision is made to act upon.

Invisible hand

Adam Smith, a well-known economist, penned the words "the invisible hand" in the 1700s. They later became the catchcry of the economic world and frequently used in the world of psychology as well.

The concept of the invisible hand has to do with the reasons behind our buying behaviour: why we buy what we do and how it equates to our economic activity, productivity and the greater economy as a whole. Our reasoning is what drives our decision-making, and I would like to suggest that our decisions are normally influenced by vice or virtue. Pursuing vice or virtue determines our path in life.

The invisible forces of good and evil drive us along. Our soul is the seat of decision regarding which path we should follow: one leads to death (vice), while the other leads to life (virtue). Suffice it to say, God gifted us with free will, so we can choose our path at any time.

Change of Governor

Why is the soul so important? Because there is a battle for your soul—and within your soul. Two opposing spiritual forces seek to influence your will, and in doing so, determine how the Central Bank of your Human Bank operates. These forces are light and darkness, good and evil—God and the devil. Look what the Bible says in Galatians 5:16-17:

"But I say, walk by the Spirit, and you will not gratify the desires
of the flesh. For the desires of the flesh are against the Spirit, and
the desires of the Spirit are against the flesh, for these are opposed
to each other, to keep you from doing the things you want to do."
Galatians 5:16–17

This scripture clearly shows the two opposing forces in the battle: the flesh,
representing our sinful nature and desire for evil, and the Spirit of God,
representing all that is good and right.

God seeks for us to surrender our will to Him. To trust God to lead and
guide us by His Spirit, the Holy Spirit. The Holy Spirit desires to lead and guide
us in truth, love, and peace, in paths of life and light.

In contrast, the devil wants not only to influence our soul but also to take
over as Governor. The devil wants control over our soul (Central Bank) so he
can govern our will, desires, thoughts, behaviours and investments into our
Human Bank, enslaving us with fears and addictions. A significant distinction
between God and the devil is that God does not seek to override our free will,
only the devil does. God gifted us our free will and lets us make our own
decisions. God's will for us is that we willingly seek Him, His Will, His Help,
His empowerment, His leading and guidance. He always guides us into love
and truth. God has a plan and purpose for all of humanity, indeed, for all of
His creation.

The devil on the other hand doesn't care about our choice, our free will, or
our wellbeing. He wants to dominate us, and he'll do it by means of tempting
us, luring us under his control and into making negative investments into our
Human Bank. Why?

When we submit to his temptations and pleasures, we become ensnared by
them and those desires start to dominate us. Trapped by them, we gradually
surrender our will, our desires, our thoughts, bit by bit, until the darkness (the
devil) takes over the Central Bank and our soul is influenced by this new
governor, with his dark will and desires. So many people around the world are
snared in darkness; addictions, loss of self and control, fear. In other words,
they have lost their freedom.

When we feel like we are starting to lose control of our mind, our will and
desires become darker; life becomes darker. That is a sure sign that the evil one
is trying to take over as governor of the central bank: our soul!

Chapter 18: Vice & Virtue

The idea of virtue and vice— or right and wrong— is not a new concept. Ancient philosophers such as Aristotle and Plato, who lived in the 4th and 5th Century BC, grappled with these often-complex theories and concepts. The role of our soul is to guide us in virtuous living, to maintain goodness, and a character that expresses and experiences love, joy, peace and hope.

Definition of Vice: Depravity or corruption of morals; evil, immoral, or wicked habits or conduct; indulgence in degrading pleasures or practices.

Definition of Virtue: Moral excellence; goodness; righteousness. Conformity of one's life and conduct to moral and ethical principles; uprightness; rectitude.

> "Virtue does not come from wealth, but wealth and every other good thing which men have comes from virtue." – Plato

In contrast, vices want to ensnare us. They replace love, joy, peace, hope, kindness and goodness with emotions, thoughts, decisions and behaviours that are negative, such as: guilt, shame, greed, lust, negative self-worth, rejection, anger etc. It is encouraging to know that you can overcome those urges and strong temptations.

> "The unexamined life is not worth living." – Socrates

When we were born, we had pure consciences. However, over time it can be corrupted by the ways of the world. Indulging in vices, things that are immoral, dark, or evil, invests the dark nature of those vices into us, changing the desires of our soul from good to bad.

> "The soul becomes dyed with the colour of its thoughts." – Marcus Aurelius

Classic Seven Deadly Vices (Seven Deadly Sins)

You may have heard of "The Seven Deadly Sins" 23. They are a concept that has been around for centuries, and the destructive effects that have wrought on humanity have been around even longer. These vices have often been recognised over the centuries as the root of moral corruption.

Vice	Effect on the soul
Wrath (Anger)	Steal peace deposits continuous anger and hate.
Greed	Steals contentment and deposits insatiable, endless and unsatisfied desires.
Gluttony	Steals self-control and deposits unrelenting cravings and desires for pleasure.
Lust	Steals love and purity Deposits false love, debauchery unrelenting selfish sexual thoughts and desires.
Sloth (Laziness)	Steals purpose and meaning deposits despondency, meaninglessness and depression.
Pride (Ego, Arrogance)	Steals connection and relationships deposits disconnection, isolation, discord.
Envy	Steals identity, meaning, self-worth deposits, discontent, rivalry, insecurity, inadequacy, deficiency.

How Vices Destroy the Soul

- They create addiction – we get enslaved to the desires.
- They cloud judgment – of what is right and wrong, good and bad.
- They disconnect from virtue –a disconnect from our True Self.
- They enslave the mind – trapping a person in self-destructive, dominating thought patterns.
- They steal - life, peace, contentment, identity, meaning and hope.

Michael J. Smith

Investment Strategy Solution

Positive investments strengthen the soul (the Central Bank of the Human Bank), increase the energy, joy, love, peace, and freedom currencies. Negative investment weakens the soul, deducting energy, joy, love, peace and freedom.

When the soul is strong it can resist vice and temptation, but when it is weak it has little defence against vices.

"The greatest victory is to conquer yourself." – Plato

The soul is our conscience, designed to guide us to paths of life, peace and fulfilment. However, we face temptations that lure us to defile and destroy our soul. These have the potential to corrupt, poison and damage our soul. Our lives will produce the fruit of what we invest in, whether dark or light, bad or good.

Conscience contains the word "science", which comes from the Latin word "Scientia", meaning, "state or fact of knowing; what is known, knowledge (of something)." So, our soul includes our intellect, our mind. It perceives and knows.

"You don't have a soul. You are a soul. You have a body." – C. S. Lewis

Our soul, the spiritual part of us, includes a conscience which is there to guide our thoughts, beliefs and actions. Its function is to protect our soul from being damaged, defiled, corrupted and overtaken. To guard the love, peace, joy, goodness and freedom. To guard the moral purity of our soul so that it springs forth life, peace, joy and goodness.

Consider:

- Did you follow the guidance into what was right?

- Perhaps you went against what you knew to be right. How did you feel after?

Vices want to steal those good virtues and change the nature of our soul from light to dark. Have you noticed that people you knew changed? From nice to bad? The light of goodness and purity of our soul can dim and grow dark, cold and despondent.

When people change it is often because of what they have allowed or inverted darkness into their life. Their soul's nature is changed into darkness

138

and negativity has taken over. That new nature now governs their soul and their Central Bank. Who Is the Governor of your soul, your Central Bank? Vice or virtue, immorality or morality, darkness or light, evil or good?

The Thief

The Enemy of Our Soul

Whether we like it or not, and believe it or not, there is an enemy of our soul.

> "The thief comes only to steal and kill and destroy. I [Jesus] came that they may have life and have it abundantly." - John 10:10

Who is the thief? The devil, or Satan (meaning "Adversary" or "Accuser" in Hebrew), is the spiritual thief that comes to **steal** our life wellbeing. If he can steal from us, he will try to **kill** us. He also seeks to **destroy** us, our health and our wellbeing, physically, emotionally, relationally, mentally, and spiritually. **In essence, the devil wants to take over as Governor of your Human Bank.**

The truth is that the enemy's goal is separation. Satan's main purpose is to separate us from Truth, God and each other. To separate us from God's truth, life, joy, love, peace, freedom. For us to hate God and to hate each other. If he can separate us from God and each other, he can separate us from truth, joy, love, peace and freedom. If he can keep us separated from God, he can keep us under his control and carry out his mission to cheat, kill and destroy us.

The devil operates through deceptions designed to lead us away from the truth about God so that we don't turn to God and receive all He wants to be and do for us. Satan uses lies to:

- Distort God's character so you don't trust Him.

- Twist your identity so you don't know who we are.

- Steal your hope, joy, and peace by making you believe you're alone and worthless.

> "When he lies, he speaks out of his own character, for he is a liar and the father of lies."- John 8:44

The Devil's Mission Versus God's Heart

Satan knows that if he can...

- Keep us away from God's truth,

- Cut us off from God's love,

- And separate us from God's life,

...then he can keep us under his control — confused, deceived, and defeated.

The Truth of God	The truth about the devil
- God loves you	- The devil hates you
God wants to give you:	**The devil wants to give you:**
- Love	- Hate
- Peace	- Anxiety
- Joy and hope	- Sadness, depression and hopelessness
- Acceptance and belonging	- Rejection and isolation
- Freedom	- Enslavement in addictions and darkness
- Truth that sets you free	- Imprisonment with lies and deceptions that separate you from life in God

• God wants us to love and forgive each other	• Hatred, conflict, unforgiveness and anger towards others
• God offers forgiveness in Jesus	• Condemnation and blame

Why we need God:

- To be **delivered** from evil.
- To be **healed** from deception.
- To be **protected** from darkness.
- To be **restored** into relationship.
- To have **spiritual life** and **freedom.**

"He has delivered us from the domain of darkness and transferred us to the kingdom of his beloved Son." Colossians 1:13

Love and Forgiveness

As stated in the table above, God wants to give us love and forgiveness. Why? God IS love, and He desires that we receive His love and love each other. We are all created in His image and likeness; we are special.

Love is called the Great Commandment in the Bible:

"Teacher, which is the great commandment in the Law?' [37] And he said to him, 'You shall love the Lord your God with all your heart and with all your soul and with all your mind. This is the great and first commandment. [3]And a second is like it: You shall love your neighbour as yourself. On these two commandments depend all the Law and the Prophets." Matthew 22:36-40

In this passage, Jesus taught us the most important things that God wants us to do:

1. Love God with all your **heart** and with all your **soul** and with all your **mind**.
2. Love neighbour as yourself.

Why Love?

God wants love to rule in our hearts, our minds, our souls and for us to be committed, purposeful in loving Him above all and loving each other. We must be committed to love above all else, because it is God's design and purpose for all of humanity. Love is not just a belief, but something that we do. Imagine:

- What would the world be like if we loved one another?
- How our lives would be different by loving God?
- What it would feel like to be full of love?

Satan knows the power inherent in loving God and each other. It hinders and stops his work of destruction, division, hate, anger, and bitterness. Satan's will is to do the opposite of all the good that God desires.

The Hurt

Satan's objective for humanity is for us to hurt each other, physically, emotionally, relationally, mentally and spiritually. And for us to not forgive each other so we are trapped in our woundedness, bitterness and upset.

Every person has had wrong done against us, sometimes great harm and injustice. I have experienced pain, injustice, rejection, and betrayal, often by those that were closest and meant to love me the most, and I'm sure this is the case for many readers. However, I have also experienced the power of forgiveness, which releases me from the past and projects me into the future.

There is a way through hurt, bitterness, and rejection, even though Satan would like the person who suffered hurt to hold onto unforgiveness. Unforgiveness is like bottling the offense in an invisible time capsule and storing it in our soul. It leads to hurt, upset, anger, bitterness. Our souls are poisoned with those bitter fruits. Our souls become angry, bitter, hurt, dark, wounded things and we now act and live out of that corrupted place. The result is that we are increasingly angry, bitter, easily upset or offended.

Perpetuation: The Great Transfer

If we have unforgiveness, Satan wants to continue the cycle of destruction, provoking us to act out of our upset by getting revenge on the perpetrator or anyone that upsets us.

And so, Satan's cycle of destruction continues, rippling out from one person to the next, often to our loved ones. We are snappy, easily triggered and react in anger; we are simply transferring all that hurt and upset onto them and others. In doing so, we advance Satan's goal of the mass global transference of hurts, upsets, anger, revenge and darkness. His desire is for those things to reign in our hearts, souls, and minds, harming ourselves, our family, friends, workplaces, communities and nations.

It could be considered a chain reaction of destruction across the nations, resulting in darkness reigning in our hearts, soul and minds. And it all started with unforgiveness.

The Soul Prison

Unforgiveness is the prison of the soul. It stops us from loving, it stops us from being loved and if we stop being loved we have the opposite: hate. We hate God and each other, thinking God doesn't love me, nobody loves me.

When we are hurt, we hurt others (even unintentionally), and tend to isolate ourselves, feeling alone and as though no one cares. If we believe God doesn't love us, we will think He doesn't care, that He doesn't do anything. In essence:

- God is hindered whilst we have unforgiveness.
- God gives us free will.
- We have free will – we have choice to hurt or to forgive.
- Others may use their free will negatively against us.
- However, we have free will to forgive.
- God doesn't force us to forgive or love.
- But unforgiveness makes that decision for us.
- We cannot love when we have unforgiveness.
- We cannot receive love when we have unforgiveness.

Unforgiveness blocks our ability to receive love and give love. It is like a wall that stops God's love from entering.

For God's love and unforgiveness cannot coexist: it's one or the other. When we have unforgiveness we are choosing destructive fruits: anger, hate, bitterness, revenge, darkness, depression, oppression. **Unforgiveness gives Satan access, influence and control in our lives and it destroys us from the inside out, like poison corroding the soul.** Does anyone truly want that?

Forgiveness

God gave us another way, and it is the path of forgiveness. Some readers may react to that comment by thinking, *You don't know what they did to me*, or *You expect me to forgive after the evil they did? How is that right?*

Those responses, and similar thoughts, are understandable. I don't know what you have been through, or what people have done to you. But I do know the way out!

The way out of the prison of pain, torment and suffering is forgiveness. Freedom comes from letting go of those hurts, upsets, or offenses, by choosing to forgive that person or persons.

Forgiveness means coming to a place where you don't have to stay in that prison. You now have a key in your hand, a key of forgiveness, that unlocks the prison doors so that you can come out into the light of freedom, liberation into love and peace.

God sent His Only Son Jesus to die for you, I and all of humanity. Because our wrongs (our sin) separated us from God, He had to forgive us so we can be united with Him.

- It was God's ultimate expression of forgiveness.
- Jesus died to pay the price for everything that we have ever done wrong (or will do).
- Jesus died for every time we have hurt someone
- Jesus died for every time we hurt, grieved and spat in the face God.

In the Bible Jesus says:

> "Truly I tell you, whatever you did for one of the least of these brothers and sisters of mine, you did for me." Matthew 25:40

In the context of the story Jesus was saying what good people have done to others, they did to Him.

> "He will reply, 'Truly I tell you, whatever you did not do for one of the least of these, you did not do for me." Matthew 25:45

Conversely, Jesus said in the above verse that whatever good that people did not do to others, they also did not do it for Him. Jesus was identifying himself with humanity, saying that whatever we do to each other, whether good or bad, we are doing the same to Jesus. In other words, we are either wounding Jesus by our actions and behaviour toward each other or blessing and loving Him by our actions and behaviour to each other.

Jesus demonstrated His love for us by dying as a sacrifice for our sins, once and for all.

> "But when Christ had offered for all time a single sacrifice for sins, he sat down at the right hand of God." Hebrews 10:12

In this way, God offered us forgiveness even when we didn't deserve it. Jesus' death was an expression of God's love and forgiveness.

> "For if while we were enemies we were reconciled to God by the death of his Son, much more, now that we are reconciled, shall we be saved by his life." Romans 5:10

God initiates and offers forgiveness so we could be reconciled back to God, united with Him. It is true forgiveness from God that we didn't deserve, and it is up to the individual to receive it.

How do we receive God's forgiveness?

- We acknowledge that we have sinned (done wrong) firstly to God and then to others.

- We thank God for sending Jesus, His Son to die for the punishment of our sin.

- We thank God for His forgiveness and that our soul can be cleansed of our wrongs and be united back to God.

As we receive that forgiveness by acknowledging to God that we have wronged God and others, God can make things right in our lives. Now, we can be free from Satan's torment; free from bonds of unforgiveness, darkness, hate, evil, and bitterness. As God forgave us, we can forgive others. Fully, not half-heartedly.

Here's a way you can exercise forgiveness right now: Say out loud: "[Name of person] I forgive you for all you did to me. Today I go free from it. What you did to me no longer has claim, power or influence over me. I forgive as God forgave me."

You CAN forgive with God's help. When you receive God's forgiveness first, it empowers you to forgive others. Why? Because God's forgiveness releases us from the bonds of darkness that held us, and we are empowered by love to forgive. As we have been forgiven and forgive others, the power of Satan is broken and we like a bird fly free.

Conditional forgiveness

> "For if you forgive others their trespasses, your heavenly Father will also forgive you, 15 but if you do not forgive others their trespasses, neither will your Father forgive your trespasses."
> Matthew 6:14-15

If we don't forgive, God our Heavenly Father cannot forgive us. This is because we are forgiven not just for ourselves but so we can forgive others. That is the ultimate purpose of God's love and forgiveness. It is not so that we can be loved and forgiven by God and then have unforgiveness and hate toward others and God. No, receiving God's love and forgiveness enables us to love and forgive others.

That is when Satan's cycle of destruction is broken and we can be restored back to the love of God, love for each other and experience the freedom of forgiveness – life and peace in our soul.

Unforgiveness is like poison to our soul. If our wellbeing is like a tree, unforgiveness withers and kills its leaves, fruit, and branches all the way down to the roots– roots of bitterness. It poisons us from the inside out.

Love and forgiveness are what our soul needs, so our wellbeing tree is nourished, growing and flourishing in the fullness of life.

Love Your Enemies

> "You have heard that it was said, 'You shall love your neighbour and hate your enemy.' But I say to you, Love your enemies and pray for those who persecute you" Matthew 5:43-44

The Fruit of Forgiveness

Fruit of Forgiveness	Fruit of Unforgiveness

Love	Anger, hate, bitterness
Joy	Resentment and revenge
Peace	Crippled by wounds and upset
Hope	Constant negative emotions, thoughts and upsets
Freedom	Captive to hurts and pains
	Steals love, joy, peace, hope, freedom, and our future

The Fruits of Unforgiveness

What happens when we choose not to forgive— physically, emotionally, relationally, mentally, and spiritually?

Bank	Fruit of Unforgiveness	Scripture
Physical Bank	Stressed restless, sleep disturbance, fatigue, high blood pressure.	"A tranquil heart gives life to the flesh, but envy makes the bones rot." Proverbs 14:30
Emotional Bank	Bitterness, resentment, anger, chronic stress, emotional numbness, trauma.	"Let all bitterness and wrath and anger and clamour and slander be put away from you... forgiving one another, as God in Christ forgave you." Ephesians 4:31–32

Relational Bank	Broken trust, isolation, ongoing conflict, hurt overtakes ability to love.	"If you do not forgive others their trespasses, neither will your father forgive your trespasses." Matthew 6:15
Mental Bank	Continuous negative thinking, anxiety, lack mental clarity, loss of peace.	"For the anger of man does not produce the righteousness of God." James 1:20
Soul Bank	Separation from God, spiritual blockage & bondage, hardness of heart prevents receiving love.	"But if you do not forgive, neither will your Father who is in heaven forgive your trespasses." Mark 11:25

Unforgiveness feels like power or protection, but it imprisons the soul. It poisons your emotional system, damages your relationships, clouds your thoughts, and keeps you spiritually stuck. It's Satan's trap to keep your Human Banks in debt. However, forgiveness opens the way for restoration, healing and replenishing of your soul.

A person cannot have true wellbeing if they have unforgiveness. Unforgiveness steals a person's wellbeing. It bankrupts them physically, emotionally, relationally, mentally, and spiritually.

The Fruit of Forgiveness

What happens when we choose to forgive— physically, emotionally, relationally, mentally, and spiritually?

Bank	Fruit of Forgiveness	Scripture
Physical Bank	Improved health, better sleep, lower stress, strengthened immunity.	"A joyful heart is good medicine, but a crushed spirit

		dries up the bones." Proverbs 17:22
Emotional Bank	Peace, release from bitterness, emotional healing, joy restored.	"Be kind to one another, tender-hearted, forgiving one another, as God in Christ forgave you." Ephesians 4:32
Relational Bank	Reconciliation, deeper love, restored trust, unity.	"Above all, keep loving one another earnestly, since love covers a multitude of sins." 1 Peter 4:8
Mental Bank	Clarity, reduced anxiety, freedom from repetitive toxic thoughts, mental peace.	"You will keep him in perfect peace whose mind is stayed on you, because he trusts in you." Isaiah 26:3
Soul Bank	Spiritual freedom, closeness with God, spiritual growth, inner peace, love and life.	"Forgive, and you will be forgiven… For with the measure you use, it will be measured to you." Luke 6:37-38

Summary

Forgiveness is not weakness; it is **spiritual strength in action**. It unblocks the flow of life to your Human Banks. Forgiveness frees you, heals you, and reconnects you with God's love, peace, and power. It fills what bitterness tried to drain. It replenishes your soul.

Forgiveness is a divine transaction — you release yourself, someone, and God releases you.

As we receive God's love and forgiveness, we can love and forgive others and the cycle of God's love and forgiveness perpetuates, rippling across our families, friends, workplaces, communities and nations.

As we love God with all our heart, soul and mind there is no room left for unforgiveness bitterness, or darkness, only love. As we love God with all our heart, soul, mind and love our neighbour as ourselves, we experience:

- Peace with God
- Peace with ourselves
- Peace with our neighbour
- Peace in our world.

The Two Streams of Love and Unforgiveness.

Loving	Unforgiveness
Love flows like a stream, watering your soul, bringing flourishing and fullness of life.	Blocks the flow of love, preventing you from giving or receiving love. Your heart and soul become dry, barren, brittle and hard.
⇓	⇓
Fruit	**Fruit**
Produces the fruits of patience, kindness, goodness, joy, peace, freedom, energy, vitality, purpose and potential.	Produces destructive behaviours to ourselves and to others: • Destructive thoughts and emotions, leading to destructive outworkings of our thoughts and emotions. • Destructive internal coping methods to cope with pain and upset - drinking, smoking, excessive media, escape etc. • Destructive external methods: anger, bitterness, resentment, violence, rage, revenge etc.
⇓	⇓

Compound Effect	**Compound Effect**
We love and forgive others. We create a new cycle of love and forgiveness.	These compound into greater negative thoughts & emotions- guilt, shame, condemnation, regret etc that can lead to unforgiveness of self for the things we have done. This exacerbates our negative behaviours, and the cycle continues.

Two Types of Unforgiveness

We can experience the effects of double unforgiveness:

- **Unforgiveness toward others** for what they did to us; this is more of an external working of upset towards others.
- **Unforgiveness to ourselves for** what we did. This is more of an internal condemnation; regret, damaged self-worth, identity leading to depression.

When we experience both forms of unforgiveness it debilitates, destroys and depletes our life physically, emotionally, relationally, mentally and in our soul. If our souls were made of clay, unforgiveness removes the moisture from the clay, making it hard and inflexible.

How Satan works

In twenty plus years of serving and supporting people, I have seen firsthand the destruction Satan brings but experience has also taught me how he operates and I would like to share some of that with you. Because Satan is stealing from your life, from your family, your friends, in workplaces in our community, and we need to be aware of his strategies.

1. Satan deceives us; he distorts truth about what really happened.
2. Satan causes conflict and strife through lying, giving us negative thoughts about other people and what they did.
3. Satan's goal is that we blame and judge other people, becoming angry with them.
4. Then, we act against them.

Ultimately Satan plants negative thoughts, lies and deceptions, about people and situations to empower us to conflict, strife, division, accusations, judgement, offense, anger, etc.

Evil strategies:

- Lies & Miscommunication

- Pride & Offense

- Assumptions & Accusations

- Unforgiveness

- Division & Gossip

- Anger & Rage

- Fear & Insecurity

Sadly, Satan has been stealing much from us, and we need to be aware that negative and destructive thoughts about others or ourselves are most likely from one source: evil. They are intended to bring destruction to our relationships and our soul. When we feel hate, rage, judgement, bitterness, offense, or unforgiveness you can be sure the author behind it is Satan. Perhaps knowing the ultimate source or our hurts and upsets may help us forgive.

It's time we stopped functioning as his instruments of destruction in the perpetuation of darkness and evil and became instruments of forgiveness, reconciliation, love and peace.

How God Fills Our Human Banks vs. How Satan Steals from Them

Physical Bank (Energy)

God Fills Through...	Satan Steals Through...
Strength by His Spirit (Ephesians 3:16).	Exhaustion from overwork & poor boundaries.

Wisdom for rest and health.	Addictions that drain energy.
Self-control from the soul.	Neglect of physical wellbeing.
	Independence (self-reliance).

Emotional Bank (Joy)

God Fills Through...	Satan Steals Through...
Joy in His presence (Psalm 16:11).	Depression, sadness, isolation.
Emotional healing.	Emotional trauma & rejection.
Hope for the future.	Lies negative thoughts & condemnation.
	Hopelessness and despair.

Relational Bank (Love)

God Fills Through...	Satan Steals Through...
Unconditional love from God (Romans 5:5).	Bitterness & unforgiveness.
Forgiveness & belonging.	Rejection & abandonment.
Healthy relationships.	Hate, anger, conflict and strife.
	Unhealed wounds and hurts.

Mental Bank (Peace)

God Fills Through...	Satan Steals Through...
Peace that surpasses understanding (Philippians 4:7).	Anxiety, confusion, fear.
Truth that renews and clears the mind.	Lies that torment.
Trust in God that gives peace.	Information overload, distraction.

Soul Bank (Freedom)

God Fills Through...	Satan Steals Through...
Freedom in Christ (John 8:36).	Bondage to sin, guilt, shame.
Purpose, identity, and eternal hope.	Identity distortion & confusion.
Light instead of darkness.	Spiritual deception & temptation.
Truth (John 8:32).	Pleasures and poor coping methods.

Summary

- **God fills** our Human Banks with life, truth, love, peace, and power through a relationship with Him.
- **Satan steals** from our Human Banks through lies, fear, temptation, and separation from God.

What is condition of your Soul your Central Bank? You will know by our fruit. What fruit are you experiencing? Energy, Love, Joy, Peace, Hope, Freedom, Goodness, Gentleness? Or negative emotions and thoughts, and experiencing: burnout, confusion, guilt, shame, pride, poor identity, poor self-worth, rejection, envy, sadness, hopelessness, despair?

"What does it profit a man to gain the whole world, but lose his soul?" – Jesus." (Mark 8:36)

Our soul can be taken over by darkness and this life. If we lose our soul, we lose our freedom.

A New Path, a New Way

"True happiness is found in the soul, not in external things." – Plato

Whatever our situation, there is hope for freedom from guilt, shame, hurts, upsets, lust, greed, anger, etc. We can start anew. Our souls are spiritual and the only way for them to be cleansed and purified is with the source of all life, goodness, purity, love and truth and power: that is, God.

God is the only one that can cleanse us from all our wrongs, making us spiritually clean. He can take away the burdens of our darkness, our guilt, our shame and restore us back to purity, wholeness, goodness, love, peace and joy.

"Let us draw near to God with a sincere heart and with the full assurance that faith brings, having our hearts sprinkled to cleanse us from a guilty conscience and having our bodies washed with pure water." Hebrews 10:22 (New International Version)

The Tale of a Man, The Tale of a City

Once upon a time there was a city, and in it lived a man named Tom.

He was a simple man; he lived by himself, and that's how he spent most of his time. Tom was somewhat of a recluse. His parents had disowned him as a child, leaving him an orphan, and he lacked education and opportunity.

Despite this, Tom was determined to make life happen and live a worthwhile life. The city promised much but delivered very little, so he set his sights beyond.

During the day he often walked along the river bank, skimming stones on the river's smooth surface and watching the ripples spread outward. *The ripple always spreads*, Tom thought. *What if my life was like a ripple that spread across the whole river? That would be special.*

Tom wanted to be different, to make an impact on people's lives that would inspire them in turn. What if he were famous throughout the city? What if people showered him with applause, accolades, instead of ignoring him? He wondered what it would be like to command an audience, to be a powerful presence on a stage.

What a day that would be, Tom thought wistfully, *Being a 'somebody' and not a 'nobody'. I would have purpose, fame and I guess fortune, too.*

Tom's vision of fame had prompted him to take action. He enrolled in acting and singing school, practising, practising. He was given a part in a local play and worked day and night to memorise his lines. A casual thought about being popular and well-known morphed into a full-blown obsession that dominated his waking hours. He could see it in his mind: the lights, the cameras, the cheering audiences.

On the route between Tom's home and the studio, he often rehearsed lyrics and recited lines, preparing for his grand performance. The neighbours, witnessing Tom's transformation from shy introvert to boisterous performer, wondered if he had received a personality transplant.

One day, Tom woke up to his phone ringing. The call was from a lady saying she was his mother. Tom could scarcely believe it. He paced the dimly light room, his thoughts racing. Confusion, anger, happiness, and sadness warred within him. Eventually Tom burst out his front door and ran down the street, shouting, "No! This can't be happening!"

Today was his big day, his first solo performance on stage. He couldn't believe it. How could this woman want to walk back into his life right at this moment? It was distraction Tom hadn't anticipated.

Nevertheless, Tom met with the woman, who vowed tearfully to make up for the lost years. Sadly, it didn't last. Like a wind blowing in one window and out the other, she disappeared from Tom's life as quickly as she had appeared. Her motivation for returning had been the guilt and shame she felt for abandoning Tom as a child, but she hadn't counted the cost of being united with him again.

Tom was devastated, but he was determined to move on, to find the love he craved in the approval of an audience. The desire for fame was still fresh in his mind and he pushed on in his relentless pursuit of notoriety.

His first performance was a success. What a buzz it created! His name was plastered across the local newspapers. People wanted to meet him; women started noticing him. He had gone from invisible to celebrity. It was like Tom had been injected with an overdose of ego and wow, it felt good. He came to crave the attention that came with performance.

It wasn't long before the national press got wind of Tom's extraordinary talent and projected him to the national spotlight. Life became a whirlwind of media interviews, shows, dressing rooms, and makeup. He indulged in every pleasure imaginable and ones that weren't.

I longed for a day when I was real to people, and now I'm living the dream, Tom thought happily. He could scarcely keep up with the pleasures; the tastes, touches, smells and sights. His senses were in overdrive, as was his libido.

Unfortunately, Tom came to learn that his lifestyle and the fame and fortunate associated with it had a cost. Sleep became less and less, as the partying and pleasures became more and more. He grew increasingly weary, but Tom wanted to make the most of it.

One day it all came crashing down. Tom learnt the hard way that drinking alcohol, smoking, sleeping around and playing gigs most nights, takes its toll on the body. Tom crawled out of bed one morning and stumbled to the bathroom, where he vomited up the night before. The gloss of lights was fading, the sound of the cheering distant as the curtain closed on my final performance.

As he regarded his haggard reflection in the mirror, Tom realized that in trying to find his way, he had become even more lost. *Now I'm not sure where I am.*

Feeling lost and overwhelmed, Tom stumbled out into the street. "Can anyone help me?" he asked. Nobody understood, pointing back to his house and saying he knew where he lived.

Tom wasn't looking for home. He was looking for peace. He vaguely recalled that he had some measure of peace as a 'nobody' before he wanted to be a 'somebody'. How he longed to get back there, to reclaim some measure of peace!

He roamed the streets of the city, searching for the path to peace. It has to be here somewhere. *The river,* he thought suddenly. *That's where I left it.* Still weary from the partying the night before, Tom staggered with all his remaining energy toward the river. Finally, he collapsed on his hands and knees upon its bank.

"Peace, Peace where are you?" Tom called out. "God where are you, help me!"

Seconds passed, then minutes. Tom realized he had drifted asleep and awoke to discover the sun shining, trees swaying gently in the breeze, and the river flowing peacefully along its course.

What happened to me, what changed? Tom wondered. He felt that something was different. After a moment, he realized what it was. He let go of all his dreams and found peace on the shore of the river. It felt like he had found himself, and a stream of refreshing was cleansing his soul. Tom breathed out the cares of the world and breathed in the peace of the Divine.

Tom rose to his feet, feeling as light as a feather, or like a carefree, newborn in the loving arms of a parent. He just wanted to shout. He had wanted to be free and now he was! *I don't know how I am, but I know I am free!* Somehow, by leaving behind the things of the world, Tom had found peace.

The end.

Have you ever felt like Tom searching for identity and meaning? Or as though you've gained the world but lost your peace and your soul? Wherever you are in life, there is hope for change. It begins by making wise investments into your Human Bank: stopping negative investments and increasing positive ones, so you can move from loss to prosperity.

Seek to reduce the demands and the withdrawals in life and increase your deposits and investments into your Human Bank. I hope this book provides a framework for you. It will take intentionality, self-control, and persistence in guarding and investing into your Human Bank (your life). But the rewards to your wellbeing and your quality of life are worth it. Take one step each day, make one decision each day, one investment each day, and you will find yourself on the path to prospering in your Human Bank.

Chapter 19: The Prospering of the Soul

Well done!

You have made it to the final chapter.

This is the culmination of your Human Bank journey - the prospering of your soul. We can prosper materially, financially, and professionally, but there is no prosperity like that which comes from the soul. Yet, we must invest in our soul for it to prosper in true life.

Prospering of the Soul

A prospering soul filled with divine energy, joy, love, peace, and freedom through connection with God is the foundation of true wellbeing. By His Holy Spirit, God fills our soul with spiritual life, which overflows into every area, enabling both the soul and the entire Human Bank™ to truly prosper.

"For whoever would save his life will lose it, but whoever loses his life for my sake will find it. For what will it profit a man if he gains the whole world and forfeits his soul? Or what shall a man give in return for his soul?"

Matthew 16:25-26

The prospering of our soul is directly connected to the prospering of our Human Bank. Prosperity happens when we receive:

Human Bank™ True Currency

The real measure of wellbeing rooted not in money, possessions, or external success, but in spiritual life received from God that fills and overflows through each Human Bank with what we truly need:

True Divine Energy - **God gives us spiritual energy**

True Divine Joy - **God gives us spiritual joy**

True Divine Love - **God gives us spiritual love**

True Divine Peace - **God gives us spiritual peace**

True Divine Freedom - **God gives us spiritual freedom**

Michael J. Smith

These things come from connecting with God. They are greater, more valuable versions of the currency we can supply ourselves. Allow me to explain this concept in greater detail.

The True Currency of the Human Banks

In addition to receiving the currencies they are designed for (energy, joy, love, peace and freedom), each Human Bank can hold divine spiritual currencies that can only come from relationship with God through His Holy Spirit. When we invest well, we prosper. When we neglect or misuse them, we experience lack, depletion, and even spiritual bankruptcy. Let's look at the divine True Currencies mentioned above:

1. Physical Human Bank™ (Energy)
True Energy Currency comes from God. It helps us develop self-control through a healthy soul; inner discipline that enables us to make positive physical investments.

Scriptures:

> **"For God gave us a spirit not of fear but of power and love and self-control."** 2 Timothy 1:7

> **"A man without self-control is like a city broken into and left without walls."** Proverbs 25:28

2. Emotional Human Bank™ (Joy)

True Joy Currency comes from a connection with God. A spiritual relationship with God that fills us with joy that overflows into our life.

Scriptures:

> **"You make known to me the path of life; in your presence there is fullness of joy; at your right hand are pleasures forevermore."** Psalm 16:11

> **"The joy of the Lord is your strength."** Nehemiah 8:10

3. Relational Human Bank™ (Love)

True Love Currency comes from connection with God, because God IS love.

Scriptures:

> **"We love because he first loved us."** 1 John 4:19

> **"Beloved, let us love one another, for love is from God, and whoever loves has been born of God and knows God."** 1 John 4:7

4. Mental Human Bank™ (Peace)

True Peace Currency comes from trusting in God; it overcomes anxiety and fear, granting us deep inner peace.

Scriptures:

> **"You keep him in perfect peace whose mind is stayed on you, because he trusts in you."** Isaiah 26:3

> **"Do not be anxious about anything, but in everything by prayer and supplication with thanksgiving let your requests be made known to God. And the peace of God, which surpasses all understanding, will guard your hearts and your minds in Christ Jesus."** Philippians 4:6-7

5. Soul Human Bank™ (Freedom)

True Freedom Currency comes from a spiritual connection with God, bringing light to our soul and freeing us from darkness and evils such as addiction and fear.

Scriptures:

> **"So, if the son sets you free, you will be free indeed."** John 8:36

Michael J. Smith

"He has delivered us from the domain of darkness and transferred us to the kingdom of his beloved Son, in whom we have redemption, the forgiveness of sins."

Colossians 1:13-14

A Pathway to God

There is a simple, Biblical path to receiving the love of God, the forgiveness of God, the Spirit of God the Truth of God = the prospering of the Soul.

Step 1: The Love of God (The Love)

God loves us! That is why He sent Jesus to rescue us from the consequences of sin.

"For God so loved the world, that he gave his only Son, that whoever believes in him should not perish but have eternal life." John 3:16

"But God shows his love for us in that while we were still sinners, Christ died for us." Romans 5:8

Step 2: The Sacrifice of Jesus (The Gift)

Jesus gave His life to pay for our sin and restore and reconcile us back to God.

"For our sake he made him to be sin who knew no sin, so that in him we might become the righteousness of God." 2 Corinthians 5:21

"Christ also suffered once for sins, the righteous for the unrighteous, that he might bring us to God..." 1 Peter 3:18

Step 3: The Gift of the Holy Spirit (The Promise)

God now dwells within and fills believers through His Spirit, bringing life, love, light, peace, joy and spiritual freedom.

"And Peter said to them, 'Repent and be baptised every one of you in the name of Jesus Christ for the forgiveness of your sins, and you will receive the gift of the Holy Spirit." Acts 2:38

"And I will ask the father, and he will give you another Helper, to be with you forever... You know him, for he dwells with you and will be in you." John 14:16-17

Step 4: The Follower (The Purpose)

God's Spirit now dwells within us, enabling us to follow God, be like God, live for God and walk on paths of life and peace and in His purpose.

"If you abide in me, and my words abide in you, ask whatever you wish, and it will be done for you. By this my Father is glorified, that you bear much fruit and so prove to be my disciples. As the father has loved me, so have I loved you. Abide in my love." John 15:7-9

"Then Jesus said to his disciples, "Whoever wants to be my disciple must deny themselves and take up their cross and follow me. For whoever wants to save their life will lose it, but whoever loses their life for me will find it. What good will it be for someone to gain the whole world, yet forfeit their soul? Or what can anyone give in exchange for their soul?" Matthew 16:24-26

Love poured out → Jesus lifted up → The Spirit poured in

When we receive the love of God by accepting Jesus as our Saviour, we also receive forgiveness and the Holy Spirit. Only then can we experience true energy, life, true joy, true love, true peace and true freedom that truly prosper our souls. Our souls prosper because we receive true riches and eternal treasure from God.

When we receive the love of God by accepting Jesus as our Saviour, we also receive forgiveness and the Holy Spirit. Only then can we experience true energy, life, joy, love, peace, and freedom, blessings that truly prosper our souls.

Our souls prosper because we receive true riches and eternal treasure from God.

The salvation of your soul is the prospering of the soul. To prosper in the soul is to receive true riches, eternal treasure - the Holy Spirit. **Salvation is true, eternal life.**

> "Blessed be the God and Father of our Lord Jesus Christ! According to his great mercy, he has caused us to be born again to a living hope through the resurrection of Jesus Christ from the dead, to an inheritance that is imperishable, undefiled, and unfading, kept in heaven for you, who by God's power are being guarded through faith for a salvation ready to be revealed in the last time. In this you rejoice, though now for a little while, if necessary, you have been grieved by various trials, so that the tested genuineness of your faith more precious than gold that perishes though it is tested by fire may be found to result in praise and glory and honour at the revelation of Jesus Christ. Though you have not seen him, you love him. Though you do not now see him, you believe in him and rejoice with joy that is inexpressible and filled with glory, obtaining the outcome of your faith, the salvation of your souls." 1 Peter 1:3-9

> "... because God is love." 1 John 4:8

> "And without faith it is impossible to please him, for whoever would draw near to God must believe that he exists and that he rewards those who seek him." Hebrews 11:6

At 6:30 a.m. one morning I was sitting in a café in Sydney, Australia, drinking a chai tea when a man sat opposite me at the table. I said hello, and we talked for a bit. He asked what I did for work, and I told him that I was just finishing writing a book.

He worked for a global banking institution. He didn't believe in God, stating we are like ants; if God was real, why would He want anything to do with us? That is the marvellous, incomprehensible truth: He cares for us because God is love. He loves you and desires for you to be with Him in this life and for eternity.

We can look prosperous on the outside and still be bankrupt in our inner world.

I know from personal experience.

Fortunately, a prosperous soul is available for all who believe in and receive Jesus Christ.

Receiving forgiveness from God and forgiving those who have hurt or offended us, is like the light shining forth at the break of day. It is a new beginning: breaking the bonds that once held us, illuminating the soul with love, truth, and peace, and restoring us.

It is a new day one in which we no longer have to search for meaning or identity, because we have found what we were looking for: God and His love.

God has done all He can for us to turn to Him. God our creator has demonstrated His love and desire for us by sending Jesus His Son to die for us, in doing so willingly paying the price for our sin: death. By His death Jesus took away the dividing wall that once stood between us and God.

> "But when Christ had offered for all time a single sacrifice for sins, he sat down at the right hand of God…" Hebrews 10:12

Every single person now has an invitation to receive:

- **The love of God**

- **The forgiveness of God**

- **The eternal life of God**

- **The Holy Spirit of God.**

God, our Heavenly Father wants to adopt us into His family as His children. He wants His Holy Spirit, to dwell in you, bringing the fullness of God, which includes energy, joy, love, peace and freedom!

> "Beloved, I pray that you may prosper in all things and be in health, just as your soul prospers." 3 John 1:2

Invitation:

Michael J. Smith

If you have never accepted God and His Love, Jesus Christ as Saviour and the Holy Spirit these things are only one step away. You can take that step by praying the following prayer:

A Prayer to Receive God's love, and the Holy Spirit:

Heavenly Father, I want to truly receive Your love. I've just read about it, but I long to experience it. I believe that Jesus died for my sin to make a way for me to be forgiven and healed. I receive Your forgiveness. I surrender my life to You. Be the Lord of my life. I ask to be born again. Holy Spirit, dwell in me, fill me, and pour that love into my heart. Heal me. Take away all evil, every deception and every fear. I receive Your love now fully and unconditionally. I am Your child. You are my Heavenly Father. Let Your love and truth change me from the inside out. In Jesus' name. Amen.

Congratulations!

You are now a child of God through faith in God!
Your sins are forgiven. You have been washed clean by the sanctifying blood of Jesus.
The Holy Spirit now dwells within you, giving life to your body, you are a temple of the Holy Spirit.
You have received an eternal inheritance and the gift of everlasting life.

What Now?
Ask the Holy Spirit to help you know the Father, the Son, and the Holy Spirit and to reveal who you are as a child of God through daily Bible reading and prayer.
Live to love God, follow Jesus, and allow the Holy Spirit to transform you.

This will change how you think, live, and see the world.
You have become a new creation in Christ, the person God created you to be: a child of God.

Summary

Your life has value. Your soul can prosper. And God longs to fill your inner life with true riches.

Key Truths to take with you:

1. Your wellbeing is not just physical it is spiritual, emotional, relational, and mental.
   We are more than bodies we are whole beings. When one bank is depleted, the others are affected. But when the soul prospers, everything else flows from that.

2. You are the steward of your Human Bank.
   Every choice you make is either an investment or a withdrawal. You are not powerless. You can rebuild. You can choose life.

3. True wealth is not money it's Energy, Joy, Love, Peace, and Freedom.
   These currencies come not from possessions, but from *God's presence* and *wise, daily choices* aligned with truth.

4. You were created to prosper from the inside out.
   Through a living relationship with God, you can find healing, clarity, and purpose and become a wise investor of your time, thoughts, relationships, and soul.

5. You don't have to stay bankrupt.
   Jesus came to give *life that is truly life*. He restores what was lost, fills what is empty, and offers peace beyond understanding.

You are not broken beyond repair, you are loved beyond measure, and you were created to prosper in your soul.

My Declaration

Read it. Declare it. Believe it.

I am not broken beyond repair.
I am loved beyond measure.
I was created to prosper
not just in body, but in soul.

My life is a Human Bank™.
Every day, I make choices that invest or withdraw
from my wellbeing -
Physically, Emotionally, Relationally, Mentally, and Spiritually.

But I am not powerless.
With God's help, I can rebuild what was depleted.
I can heal what was hurting.
I can restore what was lost.

True riches are not found in money or status,
but in the divine currencies of:

Energy,   Joy,   Love,   Peace, and   Freedom.

And these come from a relationship with God
who fills my soul with life that is truly life.

**Today, I choose to become
a wise investor in my Human Bank™.
Today, I begin the journey of true prosperity
from the inside out.**

**This is not just a new mindset.
It's a new way to live.**

**I am currently writing the sequel to _The Human Bank - The Prospering of the Soul_.
It is planned for release in 2025, God willing!**

This next book will help you prosper in your soul, grow deeper in your faith, and walk more closely with God.
It will guide you to keep investing in your soul—the place where true life begins and flourishes.

Keep in Touch
Subscribe and follow _Human Bank_™ on social media, share your Human Bank story, and explore more resources at **www.humanbank.life**
Thank you for taking the time to read _Human Bank_.

I pray this marks the beginning of a wonderful new journey the prospering of your soul and your whole wellbeing as you walk daily with God in the life that is truly life.

For God So Loved the World

"For God so loved the world, that he gave his only Son, that whoever believes in him should not perish but have eternal life."

John 3:16

Human Bank™ Resources

Acknowledgement: Digital Research Assistance

I acknowledge the support of OpenAI's ChatGPT in the development of this book. This AI tool assisted with content structuring, research synthesis, scoring methodology, formatting, grammar, and clarity—while preserving the author's voice and message. It also supported Scripture referencing and thematic alignment between biblical truths and wellbeing principles. Final editorial decisions remain solely my own.

To utilise the Human Bank Resources, you can print off the templates, for free resources go to **www.humanbank.life** or scan the QR Code.

SCAN ME

Human Bank™ Investment Assessment

Human Bank	Positive Investment	Score: 0 Not at all - 5 Always
Physical Bank	Daily, I eat a healthy and nutritious diet (high in fruit & vegetables and low in fat, salt, sugar).	
	Daily, I experience exercise (30 - 60 mins).	
	Daily, I have self-control to avoid unhealthy coping mechanisms (e.g., excessive eating, excessive drinking, avoidance, substance use, isolation,	

	excessive screen time, media, or shopping) to deal with stress, anxiety, or negative emotions.
Emotional Bank	Each day, I heal emotional upset by processing my feelings, releasing anger, and letting go of bitterness and resentment.
	Each day, I live in alignment with my authentic 'True' self—my values, beliefs, passions, and purpose.
	Each day, I express gratitude, recognising that while I may not have everything I want or need, I am content with my life.
Relational Bank	Each day, I offer help and support to those in need in my life.
	Each day, I cultivate deep, authentic relationships with people who uplift and support me.
	Each day, I have enough money for essentials and spend my money wisely, avoiding debt.
Mental Bank	Each day, I practice forgiveness, both for others and for myself.
	Each day, I live with a sense of meaning and purpose that guides my actions.
	Each day, I trust in God with things beyond my control.
Soul (Spiritual) Bank	Each day, I experience a connection to my faith in God that brings me love, peace, and hope.
	Each day, I live to love and honour God and others with my actions.
	Each day, I dedicate time to prayer and personal Bible reading.

Human Bank	15 Negative Investments	Score: 0 (Not at all) - 5 (Always)
Physical Bank	Each day, I do not nourish my body with a balanced diet rich in fruits and vegetables while limiting unhealthy fats, salt, and sugar.	
	Each day, I do not engage in at least 30–60 minutes of physical activity to strengthen my body and improve my wellbeing.	
	Each day, I do not prioritise getting 7–9 hours of restful sleep to restore my energy and health.	
Emotional Bank	Each day, I struggle to feel safe in the workplace, online, or at home.	
	Each day, I expose myself to dark or harmful media, including violent content, coarse language, negativity, or sexualised material.	
	Each day, I engage in smoking, harming my body and long-term health.	
Relational Bank	Each day, I engage in addictive behaviours (e.g., excessive social media use, video gaming, online shopping, TV streaming, excessive working, compulsive internet use, pornography, gambling, smoking, drinking, or substance use) that feel out of my control.	
	Each day, I exhibit negative behaviours such as dishonesty, impulsivity, or destructive words and actions that harm myself and others.	
	Each day, I drink alcohol, often in unhealthy amounts (four or more drinks).	
Mental Bank	Each day, I struggle with mental health and with chronic illness challenges such as chronic pain,	

	depression, fear, anxiety, or continual negative thoughts.
	Each day, I consume excessive amounts (two or more) of caffeine or energy drinks, negatively impacting my health.
	I regularly misuse prescription or recreational drugs, affecting my wellbeing.
Soul Bank	Each day, I choose not to believe in God.
	Each day, I struggle to find meaning, hope, or purpose, leaving me feeling lost or unfulfilled.
	Each day, I find it difficult to forgive myself and others, holding onto resentment, hurt, and pain.

Positive Investment Score - Negative Investment Score = Human Bank Profit/Loss Score

Human Bank™ Profit & Loss Statement (Template)

Bank	Profitable Investments (Income)	Loss Investments (Expenses)	Net Profit/Loss
Physical			
Emotional			
Relational			
Mental			
Soul			

Total Income & Expenses		-	

Net Human Bank Balance = Profits – Losses

Now, you can implement an Investment Strategy.

Positive Investments – seek to increase your lowest rated Investments

Negative Investments – seek to decrease your highest rated Investments

Human Bank™ Investment Strategy Plan (Template)

WEEK: _____

DAILY/WEEKLY INVESTMENTS

Chose a Positive investment for each Human Bank.

Human Bank	Currency	Key Investments (List your chosen actions)	Frequency (Daily/Weekly)	Priority (1–5)
Physical Bank	**Energy**			
Emotional Bank	**Joy**			
Relational Bank	**Love**			

Mental Bank	**Peace**
Soul Bank	**Freedom**

WEEKLY REVIEW

1. What went well this week in your investments?

_____

2. Where did you feel drained or in deficit?

_____

3. What patterns or themes do you notice?

_____

4. What's one thing you'll do differently next week?

_____

WEEKLY SUPPLY & DEMAND SNAPSHOT

How much does your daily life demand and give you Human Bank Currency?

Human Bank Currency	IN Rating (0–5)	OUT Rating (0–5)	Balance (IN-OUT)	Result P+ or N – (Circle)
Physical/Energy				P or N
Emotional/Joy				P or N
Relational/Love				P or N

175

Mental/Peace				P or N
Soul/Freedom				P or N

Your Human Bank - Personalised Strategy Action Plan

This action plan is tailored to help you improve in Physical, Emotional, Relational, Mental, and Spiritual wellbeing, focusing on practical, achievable steps in each area.

Steps:

Investment Action Plan

1. **Select an investment** – Choose one positive investment you want to incorporate into your life or one negative investment you want to stop.

2. **Daily Action Plan** – Identify two or three actions that will help you either make a positive investment or eliminate a negative investment from your daily routine.

3. **Schedule Time** – Investments do not happen on their own. Dedicate time each day to take action. Once you start, you will build momentum—stay consistent and **persistent**, and you will begin to see the impact.

4. **Review Progress** – Regularly pause, reflect, and evaluate your progress.

5. **Make Adjustments** – Identify any barriers preventing you from making or stopping an investment and create solutions to overcome challenges.

6. **Keep Investing** – Continue until it becomes a routine and is fully incorporated into your life.

7. **Sustain and Expand** – Keep going until investing in your wellbeing becomes a lifestyle, and you feel empowered to make further positive investments.

Well done! You are making investments that will prosper your soul, enhance your wellbeing, and strengthen your Human Bank. Keep going!

The Human Bank™ Glossary

This glossary outlines proprietary terms within the *Human Bank*™ wellbeing framework. These definitions are rooted in original intellectual property combining biblical truth and economic principles for holistic wellbeing. All terms are protected under applicable trademark and copyright laws.

Defining Human Bank™

Physical Human Bank

Emotional Human Bank

Relational Human Bank

Mental Human Bank

Soul Human Bank

Human Bank™ Currency

Human Bank™ True Currency

Human Bank™ Investments

Positive Human Bank™ Investments

Negative Human Bank™ Investments

Human Bank™ Investment Impact

Human Bank™ Supply and Demand

Human Bank™ Supply and Demand Equilibrium

Human Bank™ Currency: Supply & Demand Index (HBCSDI)

Negative Coping Mechanisms

Human Bank™ Insolvency Bankruptcy

Central Bank of the Human Bank™

Governor *(of the Human Bank™)*

Human Bank™ Profit & Loss

Michael J. Smith

Human Bank™ Profit & Loss Statement

Human Bank™ Balance Sheet

Human Bank™ Liability

Human Bank™ Asset

Human Bank™ Return on Investment (ROI)

Human Bank™ Return on Positive Investment Model

Human Bank™ Return on Negative Investment Model

Human Bank™ Counterfeit/Foreign Currency

Human Bank™ Law of Diminishing Return

Human Bank™ Opportunity Cost

Human Bank™ Opportunity Cost Model for 15 Negative Investments - Definition

Human Bank™ Opportunity Cost Model for 15 Positive Investments

Human Bank™ Cost Benefit

Human Bank™ Investment Strategy

Prospering of the Soul

Defining Human Bank™

The Human Bank concept merges economic theory with Biblical truth within a wellbeing framework, allowing us to invest in and evaluate the profitability of our overall life wellbeing our Human Bank.

Physical Human Bank

The domain of bodily wellbeing fuelled by nutrition, exercise, sleep, and healthy self-control. It is replenished through consistent care of the body and avoiding harmful coping behaviours. **Its currency is Energy.**

Emotional Human Bank

The domain of inner emotional health strengthened by gratitude, emotional processing, self-alignment, and emotional safety. It is drained by fear, exposure to harmful media, and emotional disconnection. **Its currency is Joy.**

Relational Human Bank

The domain of healthy relationships built through generosity, trust, honesty, support, and financial responsibility. It is weakened by addictions, harmful behaviours, and relational conflict. **Its currency is Love.**

Mental Human Bank

The domain of mental clarity and resilience nourished by forgiveness, faith, meaning, and wise thought patterns. It is depleted by anxiety, substance misuse, and persistent negative thoughts. **Its currency is Peace.**

Soul Human Bank

The domain of spiritual wellbeing flourishing through faith, prayer, purpose, and connection with God. It is harmed by unbelief, lack of hope, unforgiveness, and spiritual disconnection. **Its currency is Freedom.**

Human Bank™ Currency

The essential resource each of the Five Human Banks needs to operate and flourish. Human Bank™ Currency - Energy, Joy, Love, Peace, and Freedom is deposited through positive investments and withdrawn to meet daily demands. By investing through the 15 Human Bank™ Investments, individuals replenish their Banks to sustain wellbeing and capacity for life.

Physical Human Bank Currency - Energy
Emotional Human Bank Currency - Joy
Relational Human Bank Currency - Love
Mental Human Bank Currency - Peace
Soul Human Bank Currency - Freedom

Human Bank™ True Currency

Michael J. Smith

The real measure of wellbeing rooted not in money, possessions, or external success, but in spiritual life received from God that fills and overflows through each Human Bank with what we truly need:

True Divine Energy - God gives us spiritual energy
True Divine Joy - God gives us spiritual joy
True Divine Love - God gives us spiritual love
True Divine Peace - God gives us spiritual peace
True Divine Freedom - God gives us spiritual freedom

Human Bank™ Investments

Human Bank™ Investments are the 15 Positive and 15 Negative evidence-based wellbeing actions that either contribute to or deplete the five Human Banks Physical, Emotional, Relational, Mental, and Soul.

Positive Human Bank™ Investments

The 15 Positive Investment actions that deposit life-giving value into the five Human Banks Physical, Emotional, Relational, Mental, and Soul. These investments fill and prosper your Human Bank, and build long-term wellbeing.

Negative Human Bank™ Investments

The 15 Negative Investment actions that drain, deplete, or damage the five Human Banks Physical, Emotional, Relational, Mental, and Soul. These actions withdraw value, diminish long-term wellbeing, and can lead to burnout and the eventual bankruptcy of your Human Bank.

Human Bank™ Investment Impact

An evidence-based scoring system that measures the effect of Positive or Negative Investments on the five Human Banks Physical, Emotional, Relational, Mental, and Soul. Each investment yields either a positive or negative return on overall wellbeing and contributes to the health or depletion of your Human Bank.

Human Bank™ Supply and Demand

A concept for evaluating the supply of and the demand for our Human Bank Currencies highlighting whether there is oversupply, undersupply, or equilibrium. It reveals the balance (or imbalance) between what is available in our wellbeing reserves and what is being withdrawn daily across the five Human Banks: Physical, Emotional, Relational, Mental, and Soul.

Human Bank™ Supply and Demand Equilibrium

The point at which the supply of Human Bank Currency meets the daily demand placed on a person's life indicating a state of balance. At equilibrium, the deposits (investments) into the five Human Banks -Physical, Emotional, Relational, Mental, and Soul match the withdrawals (demands), resulting in stability, sustainability, and wellbeing.

Human Bank™ Currency: Supply & Demand Index (HBCSDI)

The *Human Bank™ Currency: Supply & Demand Index (HBCSDI)* is a diagnostic matrix designed to evaluate the balance between the supply and daily demand of Human Bank Currency across the five Human Banks: Physical, Emotional, Relational, Mental, and Soul.

It helps individuals:

- Identify surplus (oversupply),

- Recognise deficit (undersupply),

- Confirm equilibrium (balanced supply and demand),

...in each Human Bank, offering insight into which domains are under strain from high demand and low supply, and highlighting where intentional reinvestment is most needed to restore wellbeing.

Negative Coping Mechanisms

Actions or behaviours that serve as negative investments into your Human Bank offering temporary relief while producing a negative return on wellbeing.

These mechanisms (e.g., pornography, substance use, or digital overconsumption) drain your Physical, Emotional, Relational, Mental, and Soul Banks, ultimately leading to depletion, imbalance, or burnout.

Human Bank™ Insolvency Bankruptcy

A critical state of depletion in which one or more of the five Human Banks - Physical, Emotional, Relational, Mental, or Soul becomes chronically drained due to repeated negative investments and insufficient replenishment. This condition often results in burnout, emotional distress, spiritual disconnection, or overall wellbeing collapse.

Central Bank of the Human Bank™

The central governing system of a person's inner life—representing the soul as the seat of identity, decision-making, and spiritual alignment. Just as a central bank regulates currency in an economy, the soul guides values, priorities, and how Human Bank Currency is invested across the five Human Banks: Physical, Emotional, Relational, Mental, and Soul.

Governor *(of the Human Bank™)*

Our Will serving as the decision-making authority that regulates how Human Bank Currency is invested or withdrawn across the five Human Banks: Physical, Emotional, Relational, Mental, and Soul. The Governor can be influenced to override the inner moral conscience our sense of right and wrong which is governed by the Central Bank of the Human Bank™: the Soul.

Human Bank™ Profit & Loss

An outcome determined by the Human Bank Investment Assessment, which evaluates whether your life is currently in profit or loss across the five Human Banks—Physical, Emotional, Relational, Mental, and Soul. It measures the net effect of your positive and negative investments to reveal whether you are replenishing or depleting your overall wellbeing.

Human Bank™ Profit & Loss Statement

A wellbeing statement that reflects the net outcome of your daily investments across the five Human Banks - Physical, Emotional, Relational, Mental, and Soul. It shows whether your overall life is in profit (growth and replenishment) or in loss (depletion and imbalance) based on your choices and behaviours.

Human Bank™ Balance Sheet

A snapshot of an individual's overall wellbeing, showing the current state of their Human Bank by comparing assets (available Human Bank Currency) to liabilities (debt or deficits in Human Bank Currency). It reflects the balance or imbalance of each of the five Human Banks: Physical, Emotional, Relational, Mental, and Soul.

Human Bank™ Liability

A negative investment, behaviour, or decision that creates a debt or burden within a person's Human Bank. Liabilities deplete Human Bank Currency across the five domains -Physical, Emotional, Relational, Mental, and Soul and reduce a person's overall wellbeing and capacity to invest positively.

Human Bank™ Asset

A positive investment, behaviour, or decision that creates Human Bank Currency (profit) within a person's Human Bank. Assets replenish and build up the Human Bank adding Energy, Joy, Love, Peace, or Freedom across the five domains: Physical, Emotional, Relational, Mental, and Soul. They enhance overall wellbeing and expand a person's capacity to invest positively.

Human Bank™ Return on Investment (ROI)

The resulting profit or loss determined through the Human Bank™ Investment Assessment. It applies evidence-based wellbeing impact to each investment across the five Human Banks - Physical, Emotional, Relational, Mental, and Soul revealing how daily choices either contribute to or diminish overall wellbeing.

Human Bank™ Return on Positive Investment Model

The **Human Bank™ Return on Positive Investment Model** reveals the evidence-based value gained from intentional, life-giving wellbeing choices. Each Positive Investment deposits Human Bank Currency—such as Energy, Joy, Love, Peace, or Freedom—into one of the five Human Banks: Physical, Emotional, Relational, Mental, or Soul.

Human Bank™ Return on Negative Investment Model

The **Human Bank™ Return on Negative Investment Model** reveals the evidence-based loss incurred from repeated unhealthy or self-damaging wellbeing behaviours. Each Negative Investment withdraws valuable Human Bank Currency—such as Energy, Joy, Love, Peace, or Freedom—from one or more of the five Human Banks: **Physical, Emotional, Relational, Mental, or Soul**.

Human Bank™ Counterfeit/Foreign Currency

Inferior substitutes for true Human Bank Currencies—external behaviours or influences that mimic value but ultimately deplete wellbeing.

• Physical Bank – Counterfeit of Energy is Stimulants
• Emotional Bank – Counterfeit of Joy is Pleasure & Entertainment
• Relational Bank – Counterfeit of Love is Pornography
• Mental Bank – Counterfeit of Peace is Substance Use
• Soul Bank – Counterfeit of Freedom is Addiction

Human Bank™ Law of Diminishing Return

A principle stating that as we use our Human Bank Currency, its return begins to diminish. When one area of Human Bank Currency (e.g., Energy, Joy, Love, Peace, or Freedom) starts to decline, it negatively impacts the others because all five Human Banks are interconnected. As one depletes, the return on investment in other areas also diminishes, reducing overall wellbeing and the profitability of the Human Bank™.

Human Bank™ Opportunity Cost

The Human Bank opportunity cost refers to the value of the wellbeing benefit lost when a person chooses one investment over another. It reflects the missed positive return that could have been gained if a more life-giving, restorative, or soul-aligned investment had been made. This impacts overall wellbeing across the five Human Banks: Physical, Emotional, Relational, Mental, and Soul.

Human Bank™ Opportunity Cost Model for 15 Negative Investments - Definition

The Human Bank Opportunity Cost Model reveals the evidence-based hidden cost of negative wellbeing investments. By choosing short-term comfort or unhealthy behaviours, individuals forfeit valuable Human Bank Currency. These lost returns such as increased Energy, Joy, Love, Peace, or Freedom represent the true opportunity cost of not making life-giving, Human Bank™ investments choices that benefit long-term wellbeing.

Human Bank™ Opportunity Cost Model for 15 Positive Investments

The Human Bank™ Opportunity Cost Model reveals the evidence-based gains unlocked through positive wellbeing investments. By choosing life-giving, restorative actions over short-term comfort or unhealthy behaviours, individuals secure valuable Human Bank™ Currency. These returns — such as increased Energy, Joy, Love, Peace, and Freedom — represent the long-term rewards of making wise, intentional choices that build lasting Human Bank™ wellbeing.

Human Bank™ Cost Benefit

Human Bank Cost-Benefit refers to the process of evaluating the personal wellbeing costs and potential benefits of a Human Bank™ investment whether Physical, Emotional, Relational, Mental, or Soul-based. It helps determine whether a choice results in a positive return (profit) or a negative return (loss) to the five Human Banks.

This model supports wiser investment decisions by weighing:

Michael J. Smith

Benefits gained - Energy, Joy, Love, Peace, Freedom
Costs incurred - Burnout, Stress, Depletion, Regret, Addiction

Human Bank™ Investment Strategy

An intentional wellbeing plan based on the 15 Positive and 15 Negative Human Bank Investments. Its goal is to increase life-giving investments that strengthen the five Human Banks - Physical, Emotional, Relational, Mental, and Soul—while decreasing negative investments that deplete or damage them. This strategy helps individuals build long-term wellbeing, spiritual alignment, and a profitable return on life.

Prospering of the Soul

A prospering soul filled with divine energy, joy, love, peace, and freedom through connection with God is the foundation of true wellbeing. By His Holy Spirit, God fills our soul with spiritual life, which overflows into every area, enabling both the soul and the entire Human Bank™ to truly prosper.

The Human Bank™ References & Research

Intellectual Property & Research Copyright Protection

The Human Bank™ Investment Framework, Methodology, and Scoring Models— including but not limited to: the Human Bank™ Return on Investment (ROI) Model, Opportunity Cost Model, Cost-Benefit Analysis (CBA), Currency Supply & Demand Index (HBCSDI), and all associated visualisations, assessments, and terminology—are original intellectual property owned by Human Bank™.

This research synthesis integrates proprietary interpretation of wellbeing domains (Physical, Emotional, Relational, Mental, and Soul), structured investment frameworks, and spiritual integration models. Any unauthorised use, reproduction, or commercial application of the content is strictly prohibited.

All referenced external sources are duly cited and acknowledged. The scoring methodology and interpretative models, while informed by published research, remain unique to the Human Bank™ system and may not be duplicated without express consent.

For permissions or licensing inquiries, contact: | www.humanbank.life

The Human Bank™ References & Research

1. Purpose of the Human Bank™ Investment Framework

The Human Bank™ Framework was developed to measure how daily behaviours act as investments either positive or negative across five domains of wellbeing:

- Physical (Energy)

- Emotional (Joy)

- Relational (Love)

- Mental (Peace)

- Soul (Freedom)

It integrates economic principles (e.g. ROI, opportunity cost), biblical truths (e.g. 3 John 1:2), and peer-reviewed health research to guide whole-life wellbeing.

2. Methodological Approach

Framework Development

- Conceptual Foundation: Merges biblical worldview with economic theory.

- Domains: Informed by spiritual formation literature and health models.

Investment Selection

- **15 Positive + 15 Negative Investments** selected from:
  - Public health
  - Psychology
  - Theology
  - Behavioural science

3. Impact Scoring Model

- **Scoring Scale**: +1 to +5 for Positive, -1 to -5 for Negative Investments.

- **Criteria**:

    1. Scientific risk/benefit level

    2. Cross-domain influence

    3. Frequency & severity in global populations

- Evidence Sources: WHO, APA, CDC, Harvard, peer-reviewed journals

4. Scoring & Assessment Tools

- ROI Modelling: Cost-benefit analysis for each investment

- Opportunity Cost: Reveals value lost when positive choices are not made

- Human Bank Currency Matrix: Maps domain impact (Energy, Joy, Love, Peace, Freedom)

5. Domain Interconnection Logic

Based on:

- Law of Diminishing Return

- Compound effect of depletion or investment in one bank on others

6. Spiritual Integration

- Biblical foundation: 3 John 1:2

- Soul Bank as central investment hub

- Flourishing requires faith, forgiveness, connection to God

7. Method Validation

Validated using:

- Anxiety/Depression indexes
- Lifestyle & risk guidelines
- Sleep, diet, exercise norms (CDC, NHS, APA)

8. HBCSDI Matrix: Supply & Demand Assessment

- Measures supply/demand of Human Bank Currency
- Ratings show surplus, deficit, or equilibrium per domain
- Data sources include: WHO, ONS UK, Mayo Clinic, Harvard, ISIC

9. Opportunity Cost Model: Negative Investments

- Measures wellbeing "forgone" due to short-term choices
- Significance Score: 0–10 based on severity, breadth, strength of correlation

10. Human Bank™ ROI Model: Negative Behaviours

- Focus: Compound negative outcomes of recurring behaviours
- Impacts: Physical, Emotional, Relational, Mental, Soul
- Return = reduction of wellbeing currency

11. Human Bank™ Cost-Benefit Analysis Framework

- Cross-domain evaluation of:
    - Daily behaviours

o Emotional/social/spiritual cost-benefit

o Return on wellbeing (Energy, Joy, Love, Peace, Freedom)

12. Core References

Includes:

- Emmons & McCullough (2003)

- Koenig (2012)

- Twenge et al. (2018)

- Walker (2017)

- Volkow, Koob & McLellan (2014)

- WHO, APA, CDC, NHS UK

This methodology enables a spiritually grounded, research-based diagnostic tool for evaluating how people invest into or deplete their total wellbeing.

Human Bank™ References & Research – Condensed Source Index

This table organises the core references and sources used across the Human Bank™ Investment Framework, grouped by topic and deduplicated for clarity.

Category	Source / Author	Publication / Organisation	Year	Notes
Physical Health & Nutrition	Harvard School of Public Health	The Nutrition Source	2021–2022	Nutrition & wellbeing
	Public Health England	Sugar Reduction Report	2019	UK dietary guidance
	NHS UK	Eat Well Guide / Activity Guidelines	2022–2023	National health standards

Category	Source / Author	Publication / Organisation	Year	Notes
	Walker, M.	Why We Sleep	2017	Sleep science & wellbeing
	Biddle & Asare	British Journal of Sports Medicine	2011	Physical activity reviews
	WHO	Global Status Reports	2018–2021	Exercise & mortality risk
Mental & Emotional Health	APA	Stress in America	2018–2023	Stress, emotions
	Emmons & McCullough	Journal of Personality & Social Psychology	2003	Gratitude & wellbeing
	Firth et al.	The Lancet Psychiatry	2020	Diet & mood science
	McEwen, B.S.	Physiological Reviews	2007	Stress neurobiology
	Sapolsky, R.M.	Why Zebras Don't Get Ulcers	2004	Chronic stress & adaptation
Spirituality & Soul Wellbeing	Koenig, H.G.	ISRN Psychiatry / Templeton Press	2012	Spiritual health
	Harvard T.H. Chan	Human Flourishing Study	2022–2023	Faith & wellbeing
	Powell et al.	Journal of Health Psychology	2003	Spiritual predictors of recovery
Addiction & Substance Use	Volkow et al.	NEJM / Brain Disease Model of Addiction	2014	Addiction neurobiology
	Koob & Volkow	Neuropsychopharmacology	2010	Reward pathways
	Grant et al.	JAMA Psychiatry	2015	Alcohol disorder stats
	Alter, A.	Irresistible	2017	Tech addiction
	Ariely, D.	The Honest Truth About Dishonesty	2012	Behavioural economics
Forgiveness, Gratitude,	Toussaint et al.	Journal of Behavioural Medicine	2016	Forgiveness & health

Category	Source / Author	Publication / Organisation	Year	Notes
Relational Health				
	Mayo Clinic	Forgiveness & Heart Health	2023	Lifestyle implications
	Ryff & Keyes	Journal of Personality & Social Psychology	1995	Wellbeing structure
Children & Adolescents Wellbeing	Twenge et al.	Clinical Psychological Science / Preventive Medicine Reports	2018	Media use & depression
Behavioural Models & CBA/ROI Methodology	WHO, CDC, NIH	Global Health Data	2013–2023	Public health impact
	APA, NHS, ONS	National Reports	Various	Mental/emotional domains

Notes:

- Duplicate entries have been consolidated under primary authors or institutions.

- References support Human Bank™'s Positive/Negative Investment Model, HBCSDI, ROI/Opportunity Cost Models, and CBA Framework.

- All scriptural integration (e.g. 3 John 1:2, Galatians 5) is from the ESV unless noted otherwise.

Footnotes

1. Human Definitions:
   o Mayr, E. (2002). *What evolution is*. Basic Books.
   o Descartes, R. (1641). *Meditations on first philosophy* (J. Cottingham, Trans., 1996). Cambridge University Press.

- The Holy Bible, English Standard Version. (2001). Crossway Bibles. (Original work published ca. 1000 BCE–100 CE)
- Maslow, A. H. (1943). A theory of human motivation. *Psychological Review*, 50(4), 370–396. https://doi.org/10.1037/h0054346
- Durkheim, E. (1893). *The division of labor in society* (W. D. Halls, Trans., 1984). Free Press.

2. Figure 1: Increase in global deaths due to NCDs and mental health (2000–2019). Source: World Health Organization (2020).

3. Figure 2: Deaths from NCDs by age group. Source: World Health Organization. (2020). *SDG Target 3.4...* https://www.who.int/data/gho/data/themes/topics/topic-details/GHO/ncd-mortality

4. Figure 3: Deaths from NCDs in those aged 30–70 years. WHO (2020). *SDG Target 3.4...* https://www.who.int/data/gho/data/themes/topics/topic-details/GHO/ncd-mortality

5. Causes of NCDs: World Health Organization. (2023). *Noncommunicable diseases: Key facts & causes.* https://www.who.int/news-room/fact-sheets/detail/noncommunicable-diseases

6. NCD Facts and Stats: WHO. (n.d.). *Noncommunicable diseases.* https://www.who.int/health-topics/noncommunicable-diseases

7. Common NCDs:
   - Campaign for Tobacco-Free Kids. (2023). *The toll of tobacco worldwide.* https://www.tobaccofreekids.org
   - CDC. (2022). *Chronic diseases.* https://www.cdc.gov/chronicdisease/index.htm
   - Encyclopaedia Britannica, Inc. (2013). *Non-communicable diseases.* https://www.britannica.com
   - NCBI. (2020). *Burden of non-communicable diseases.* https://pmc.ncbi.nlm.nih.gov/articles/PMC7124486/
   - Scientia Educare. (n.d.). *Non-communicable diseases: Lifestyle and genetic factors.* https://scientiaeducare.com
   - UNDP. (2022). *Addressing the social determinants of NCDs.* https://www.undp.org
   - World Bank. (2022). *Noncommunicable diseases overview.* https://www.worldbank.org
   - WHO. (2023). *Noncommunicable diseases: Key facts.* https://www.who.int

8. Definition of Health: World Health Organization. (1948). *Constitution of the World Health Organization.*

9. NCD Symptoms & Lifestyle Impact References:

- o WHO. (2023). *Global report on diet and health.* https://www.who.int
- o CDC. (2022). *Physical activity and chronic disease.* https://www.cdc.gov
- o WHO. (2021). *Tobacco use and disease burden.* https://www.who.int
- o NIH. (2022). *Alcohol and chronic disease study.* https://www.nih.gov
- o The Lancet. (2021). *Mental health and chronic disease link.* https://www.thelancet.com
- o WHO. (2023). *Cardiovascular disease report.* https://www.who.int
- o American Cancer Society. (2022). *Cancer facts & figures 2022.* https://www.cancer.org
- o CDC. (2021). *Chronic respiratory diseases surveillance.* https://www.cdc.gov
- o WHO. (2023). *Diabetes global report.* https://www.who.int
- o Alzheimer's Association. (2022). *Neurological disorders review.* https://www.alz.org
- o National Kidney Foundation. (2021). *Chronic kidney disease study.* https://www.kidney.org

10. Ralston, J., Brinsden, H., & Nugent, R. (2020). Global political commitment needed to tackle NCDs. *The BMJ*, 368, l4746. https://doi.org/10.1136/bmj.l4746
11. WHO. (2020). *Physical activity and health.* https://www.who.int
12. CDC. (2021). *Well-being concepts.* https://www.cdc.gov/hrqol/wellbeing.htm
13. Centers for Disease Control and Prevention (CDC). (2021). *Well-being concepts: Relational wellbeing.* https://www.cdc.gov/hrqol/wellbeing.htm
14. WHO. (2004). *Promoting mental health: Concepts, emerging evidence, practice: Summary report.* https://www.who.int/publications/i/item/9241591595
15. Koenig, H. G. (2012). Religion, spirituality, and health: The research and clinical implications. *ISRN Psychiatry*, 2012, 1–33. https://doi.org/10.5402/2012/278730
16. Encyclopaedia Britannica. (n.d.). *Supply and demand.* https://www.britannica.com/money/supply-and-demand
17. Federal Deposit Insurance Corporation. (n.d.). *When a bank fails – Facts for depositors, creditors, and borrowers.* https://www.fdic.gov/resources/resolutions/bank-failures/failed-bank-list/bank-failure-facts.html

Wikipedia contributors. (n.d.). *Bank failure*. Wikipedia.
https://en.wikipedia.org/wiki/Bank_failure

18. Investopedia. (n.d.). *Market failure*.
    https://www.investopedia.com/terms/m/marketfailure.asp
19. Investopedia. (n.d.). *Law of diminishing marginal returns*.
    https://www.investopedia.com/terms/l/lawofdiminishingmarginalre
    turn.asp
20. Wikimedia Commons. (2024). *Diminishing returns [Diagram]*.
    https://commons.wikimedia.org/w/index.php?curid=156411253.
    Licensed under CC BY-SA 4.0.
21. Economic Cost of Poor Employee Wellbeing:

    o World Economic Forum. (2020). *The Future of Jobs Report 2020*.
      https://www.weforum.org
    o Harvard Business Review. (2010). *What's the hard return on employee
      wellness programs?* https://hbr.org
    o Gallup. (2020). *State of the American Workplace*.
      https://www.gallup.com
    o American Institute of Stress. (2022). *Workplace Stress*.
      https://www.stress.org
    o WHO. (2019). *Mental health in the workplace*. https://www.who.int
    o PwC. (2018). *Experience is everything*. https://www.pwc.com
    o Gallup. (2021). *Employee Burnout: Causes and Cures*.
      https://www.gallup.com

22. Conscience Definitions:

    o Lewis, C. S. (1943). *The Abolition of Man*. HarperOne.
    o Lewis, C. S. (1952). *Mere Christianity*. HarperOne.
    o Oxford English Dictionary. (2023). *Oxford University Press*.
      https://www.oed.com/
    o Bowker, J. (Ed.). (2000). *The Concise Oxford Dictionary of World
      Religions*. Oxford University Press.

23. Catechism of the Catholic Church. (1994). *Catechism of the Catholic
    Church* (2nd ed., §1866). Libreria Editrice Vaticana.

About the Author – Michael J. Smith

Michael J. Smith lives in Sydney, Australia. He entered the business world at the age of twenty, but at twenty-three, he had a life-changing encounter with God—an experience that sparked deep inner transformation and gave him a clear sense of purpose.

For over two decades, he has devoted his life to encouraging others to invest in their wellbeing—helping people break free from burnout, stress, anxiety, depression, and darkness, and guiding them to find life in God and experience true love, joy, peace, and freedom in their soul.

The Human Bank™ is the fruit of that 20-year journey—a practical, faith-filled framework born out of lived experience, spiritual insight, and a deep commitment to whole-life wellbeing.

You can get in touch with Michael @ www.humanbank.life

Michael J. Smith